High-Yield

Genetics

High-Yield
Genetics

Ronald W. Dudek, Ph.D.
Professor
Brody School of Medicine
East Carolina University
Department of Anatomy and Cell Biology
Greenville, North Carolina

John E. Wiley, Ph.D.
Professor
Brody School of Medicine
East Carolina University
Department of Pediatrics, Clinical Genetics
Greenville, North Carolina

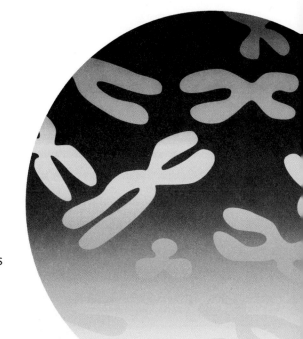

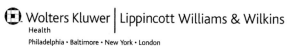 Wolters Kluwer | Lippincott Williams & Wilkins
Health
Philadelphia • Baltimore • New York • London
Buenos Aires • Hong Kong • Sydney • Tokyo

Acquisitions Editor: Betty Sun
Development Editor: Kathleen H. Scogna
Managing Editor: Kelley Squazzo
Marketing Manager: Emilie Moyer
Production Editor: Beth Martz
Design Coordinator: Terry Mallon
Compositor: Aptara, Inc.

351 West Camden Street   530 Walnut Street
Baltimore, MD 21201   Philadelphia, PA 19106

Printed in the United States of America

9 8 7 6 5 4 3 2 1

Library of Congress Cataloging-in-Publication Data

Dudek, Ronald W., 1950-
   High-yield genetics / Ronald W. Dudek, John E. Wiley.
     p. ; cm.
   Includes index.
   ISBN 978-0-7817-6877-1
  1. Medical genetics—Examinations, questions, etc. 2. Human
genetics—Examinations, questions, etc. 3. Physicians—Licenses—United States—Examinations—Study guides. I. Wiley, John E. II. Title.
   [DNLM: 1. Genetics, Medical—Examination Questions. QZ 18.2 D845h 2009]
   RB155.D83 2009
   616′.042076—dc22

                                                                  2008018887

DISCLAIMER

   Care has been taken to confirm the accuracy of the information present and to describe generally accepted practices. However, the authors, editors, and publisher are not responsible for errors or omissions or for any consequences from application of the information in this book and make no warranty, expressed or implied, with respect to the currency, completeness, or accuracy of the contents of the publication. Application of this information in a particular situation remains the professional responsibility of the practitioner; the clinical treatments described and recommended may not be considered absolute and universal recommendations.

   The authors, editors, and publisher have exerted every effort to ensure that drug selection and dosage set forth in this text are in accordance with the current recommendations and practice at the time of publication. However, in view of ongoing research, changes in government regulations, and the constant flow of information relating to drug therapy and drug reactions, the reader is urged to check the package insert for each drug for any change in indications and dosage and for added warnings and precautions. This is particularly important when the recommended agent is a new or infrequently employed drug.

   Some drugs and medical devices presented in this publication have Food and Drug Administration (FDA) clearance for limited use in restricted research settings. It is the responsibility of the health care provider to ascertain the FDA status of each drug or device planned for use in their clinical practice.

To purchase additional copies of this book, call our customer service department at (800) 638-3030 or fax orders to (301) 223-2320. International customers should call (301) 223-2300.

Visit Lippincott Williams & Wilkins on the Internet: http://www.lww.com. Lippincott Williams & Wilkins customer service representatives are available from 8:30 am to 6:00 pm, EST.

To my parents, J. Edwin "Ed" Wiley and Marie C. Wiley, whose love, support, and infinite patience allowed me to pursue my dreams.

—JOHN E. WILEY

Preface

Dr. Wiley and I are pleased to author the first edition of *High-Yield Genetics*, which marks a significant contribution to the *High-Yield* series.

Lippincott Williams & Wilkins and all of the authors of the *High-Yield* series are committed to producing books that provide a USMLE Step 1 review that not only has the breadth to cover all disciplines but also the depth of information necessary to match the question difficulty on the exam.

Since many U.S. medical schools are unable to find adequate time in the curriculum for an in-depth genetics course, medical students find themselves in a less than advantageous position when reviewing Genetics for the USMLE Step 1. A brief visit to any medical bookstore will reveal that there are about six excellent genetics textbooks that cover basic genetics and modern molecular genetic advancements. Although these are good textbooks, they are not designed for a review process under the time constraints that medical students face when preparing for the USMLE Step 1. Consequently, Dr. Wiley and I wrote *High-Yield Genetics* with the goal of placing the student in a strategic position to review genetics in a reasonable time period and most importantly to answer all of the genetics questions that would likely appear on the USMLE Step 1.

Discussions concerning the preparation for the USMLE Step 1 usually include mention of the "Big Three": Pathology, Pharmacology, and Physiology. For many USMLE Step 1 clinical case–style questions, these three disciplines coordinate nicely to present a clinical case and then ask a mechanistic question as to WHY something is observed or HOW a specific drug treatment works. The "Big Three" has become a perfect triad for USMLE Step 1 preparation.

However, in the future, we think that a "New Big Three" will develop: Embryology, Genetics, and Molecular Biology. With the completion of the Human Genome Project and the advancement of genome mapping for every individual, the future of medicine will revolve around the elucidation of the genetics of birth defects and other human diseases spearheaded by molecular biology techniques. Exactly when the "New Big Three" will have significant representation on the USMLE Step 1 is impossible for us to predict. Yet, when this does occur, the *High-Yield* series will be strategically placed to serve its customers with three superb publications: *High-Yield Embryology*, *High-Yield Genetics*, and *High-Yield Cell and Molecular Biology*. Since I (Dr. Dudek) am the common author to all three publications, I will ensure that they will be well integrated, have minimal overlap, and are updated with the latest information.

More than any other field of medicine in the future, genetics and molecular biology will be the engines that drive new breakthroughs and new information that are relevant to clinical practice. This will require that *High-Yield Genetics* and *High-Yield Cell and Molecular Biology* be routinely updated with new clinically relevant information. For this, I rely on my readers to e-mail me suggestions, comments, and new ideas for future editions: *dudekr@ecu.edu*.

Dr. Ron W. Dudek
Dr. John Wiley

Contents

6 Uniparental Disomy and Trinucleotide Repeats 32

7 Multifactorial Inherited Diseases 38

8 Mitochondrial Inheritance 47

9 Mitosis, Meiosis, and Gametogenesis 52

10 Chromosome Morphology Methods 59

Chapter 1

The Human Nuclear Genome

I. General Features (Figure 1-1)

A. The human genome refers to the haploid set of chromosomes (nuclear plus mitochondrial) that is divided into the very complex **nuclear genome** and the relatively simple **mitochondrial genome** (discussed in Chapter 8).

B. The human nuclear genome codes for ≈30,000 **genes**, which make up ≈2% **of the human nuclear genome.**

C. There are ≈27,000 **protein-coding genes** (i.e., they follow the central dogma of molecular biology: DNA is transcribed into messenger RNA (mRNA), which is then translated into protein).

D. There are ≈3,000 *RNA*-coding genes (i.e., they do not follow the central dogma of molecular biology: DNA is transcribed into RNA, which is then **NOT** translated into protein).

E. The fact that the ≈30,000 genes make up only ≈2% of the human nuclear genome means that ≈2% **of the human nuclear genome consists of coding DNA, and ≈98% of the human nuclear genome consists of noncoding DNA.**

F. The human nuclear genome contains **protein-coding genes and** *RNA*-coding genes and is under **epigenetic control** (see section IV below).

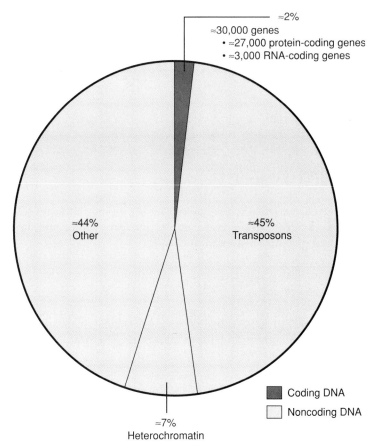

≈2%
≈30,000 genes
• ≈27,000 protein-coding genes
• ≈3,000 RNA-coding genes

≈44%
Other

≈45%
Transposons

Coding DNA
Noncoding DNA

≈7%
Heterochromatin

● **Figure 1-1** Pie chart indicating the organization of the human nuclear genome. Heterochromatin is condensed chromatin and is transcriptionally inactive (see Chapter 2, IVA).

Ⅱ Protein-Coding Genes

A. SIZE. The size of protein-coding genes varies considerably from the 1.7 kilobase (kb) insulin gene → 45 kb LDL receptor gene → 2,400 kb dystrophin gene.

B. EXON–INTRON ORGANIZATION. Exons (expression sequences) are coding regions of a gene with an average size of <200 base pairs (bp). Introns (intervening sequences) are noncoding regions of a gene with a huge variation in size. A small number of human genes (generally small genes <10 kb) consists only of exons (i.e., no introns). However, most genes are composed of exons and introns.

C. REPETITIVE DNA SEQUENCES. Repetitive DNA sequences may be found in both exons and introns.

D. CLASSIC GENE FAMILY. A classic gene family is a group of genes that exhibit a high degree of sequence homology over most of the gene length.

E. GENE SUPERFAMILY. A gene superfamily is a group of genes that exhibit a low degree of sequence homology over most of the gene length. However, there is relatedness in the protein function and structure. Examples of gene superfamilies include the immunoglobulin superfamily, globin superfamily, and the G-protein receptor superfamily.

F. ORGANIZATION OF GENES IN GENE FAMILIES.
1. **Single cluster.** Genes are organized either as a **tandem repeated array** (where one gene is repeated again and again right next to another on a single chromosome), **close clustering** (where the genes on a single chromosome are controlled by a single expression control locus), or as **compound clustering** (where related and unrelated genes are clustered on a single chromosome).
2. **Dispersed.** Genes are organized in a dispersed fashion at two or more different chromosome locations all on a single chromosome.
3. **Multiple clusters.** Genes are organized in multiple clusters at various chromosome locations and on different chromosomes.

G. UNPROCESSED PSEUDOGENES, TRUNCATED GENES, AND INTERNAL GENE FRAGMENTS. Gene families are typically characterized by the presence of unprocessed pseudogenes (i.e., defective copies of genes that are not transcribed into mRNA), truncated genes (i.e., portions of genes lacking 5′ or 3′ ends), or internal gene fragments (i.e., internal portions of genes) that are formed by **tandem gene duplication.**

H. PROCESSED PSEUDOGENES. Processed pseudogenes are transcribed into mRNA and converted to complementary DNA (cDNA) by reverse transcriptase. Then, the cDNA is integrated into a chromosome. A processed pseudogene is typically not expressed as protein, because it lacks a promoter sequence.

I. RETROGENE. A retrogene is a processed pseudogene where the cDNA integrates into a chromosome near a promoter sequence by chance. If this happens, the processed pseudogene will express protein. If selection pressure ensures the continued expression of the processed pseudogene, the processed pseudogene is considered a **retrogene.**

Ⅲ RNA-Coding Genes. RNA-coding genes produce **active RNAs** that can profoundly alter normal gene expression and hence produce an altered trait or disease.

A. 45S AND 5S RIBOSOMAL RNA (*rRNA*) GENES.
1. The *rRNA* genes encode for **rRNAs** that are used in **protein synthesis.**
2. A set of *rRNA* genes located inside the nucleolus are transcribed by **RNA polymerase I** to form **45S rRNA.** This set of *rRNA* genes is located on the short arm of five pairs of chromosomes (i.e., 13, 14, 15, 21, and 22) that contain about **200 copies** of *rRNA* genes arranged in **tandem repeated clusters.**
3. Another set of *rRNA* genes located outside of the nucleolus are transcribed by **RNA polymerase III** to form **5S rRNA.**
4. The 45S rRNA becomes associated with the 5S rRNA, ribosomal proteins, RNA-binding proteins, and small ribonucleoprotein particles (snRNPs) to form a large complex that is later split into the 40S and 60S subunits of the ribosome.

B. TRANSFER RNA (*tRNA*) GENES.
1. The *tRNA* genes encode for **tRNAs** that are used in **protein synthesis.**
2. There are 497 *tRNA* genes and 324 tRNA-derived putative pseudogenes.

C. SMALL NUCLEAR RNA (*snRNA*) GENES.
1. The *snRNA* genes encode for **snRNAs** that are components of the spliceosome used in **RNA splicing** during protein synthesis.
2. There are ≈70 *snRNA* genes that encode for **uridine-rich snRNA** (e.g., U1-U6 snRNAs), which are components of the **major GU-AG spliceosome.**

D. SMALL NUCLEOLAR RNA (*snoRNA*) GENES. The *snoRNA* genes encode for **snoRNAs** that direct site-specific base modifications in rRNA (e.g., 2'-O-ribose methylation or pseudouridylation), where uridine is isomerized to pseudouridine.

E. REGULATORY *RNA* GENES.
1. The regulatory *RNA* genes encode for **RNAs** that are likened to mRNA because they are transcribed by RNA polymerase II, 7-methylguanosine capped, and polyadenylated.
2. The **7SK** *RNA* gene encodes for **7SK RNA** that functions as a negative transcriptional regulator of RNA polymerase II elongation.
3. The **SRA-1 (steroid receptor activator)** *RNA* gene encodes for **SRA-1 RNA** that functions as a coactivator of several steroid receptors.
4. The *XIST* gene encodes for **XIST RNA** that functions in X chromosome inactivation.

F. XIST *RNA*-CODING GENE.
1. X chromosome inactivation is a process whereby either the **maternal X chromosome (X^M)** or **paternal X chromosome (X^P)** is inactivated, resulting in a heterochromatin structures called the *Barr body*, which is located along the inside of the nuclear envelope in female cells.
2. This inactivation process overcomes the sex difference in *X* gene dosage. Males have one X chromosome and are therefore **constitutively hemizygous**, but females have two X chromosomes. Gene dosage is important because many X-linked proteins interact with autosomal proteins in a variety of metabolic and developmental pathways, so there needs to be a tight regulation in the amount of protein for key dosage-sensitive genes.
3. X chromosome inactivation makes females **functionally hemizygous**. X chromosome inactivation begins early in embryologic development at about the **late blastula stage**. Whether the X^M or the X^P becomes inactivated is a **random and irreversible event**.
4. Once a progenitor cell inactivates the X^M, for example, all of the daughter cells within that cell lineage will also inactivate the X^M (the same is true for the X^P). This is called *clonal selection* and means that **all females are mosaics** comprising mixtures of cells in which either the X^M or X^P is inactivated.
5. X chromosome inactivation does not inactivate all of the genes; **≈20% of the total genes** on the X chromosome escape inactivation.

G. MicroRNA (*miRNA*) GENES (Figure 1-2A).
1. The *miRNA* genes encode for **miRNAs** that block the expression of other genes.
2. There are ≈250 *miRNA* genes with the *lin-4* **gene**, which encodes **lin-4 miRNA**, and the *let-7* **gene**, which encodes **let-7 miRNA** and is the most studied.

H. ANTISENSE *RNA* GENES (Figure 1-2B).
1. The antisense *RNA* genes encode for **antisense RNA** that binds to mRNA and physically blocks translation.
2. During protein synthesis, the DNA template strand is transcribed into mRNA (or "**sense**" RNA) from which a protein is translated. The DNA nontemplate strand is normally not transcribed. However, there are ≈1,600 genes in which the DNA nontemplate strand is also transcribed, thereby producing "**antisense**" RNA.

I. RIBOSWITCH GENES (Figure 1-2C). The riboswitch genes encode for **riboswitch RNA**, which binds to a target molecule, changes shape, and then switches on protein synthesis.

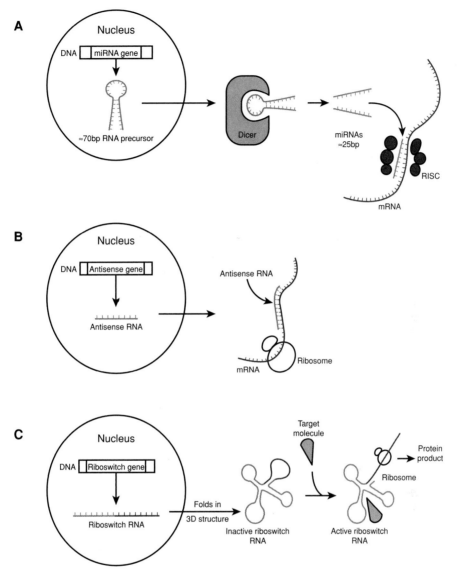

● **Figure 1-2 Some *RNA* coding genes. A:** MicroRNA genes. The *miRNA* genes are first transcribed into a ≈**70 bp RNA precursor** containing an inverted repeat that permits double-stranded hairpin RNA formation. This ≈70 bp RNA precursor is cleaved by a double-stranded RNA-specific endonuclease called ***Dicer***, which produces ≈25 bp RNA product called ***small interfering RNA* (siRNA) or *microRNA* (miRNA)**. The double-stranded miRNA unwinds to form a single-stranded miRNA, which then hunts for a matching sequence on some mRNA encoding for some protein. When the miRNA binds to the mRNA, a **RNA-induced silencing complex (RISC)** is formed, which either cleaves the mRNA or physically blocks translation. In either case, the expression of the gene that encoded the mRNA is blocked. Therefore, miRNAs seem to be very potent blockers of gene expression. (miRNA, microRNA; Dicer, double-stranded RNA-specific endonuclease; mRNA, messenger RNA; RISC, RNA-induced silencing complex.) **B:** Antisense *RNA* genes. The antisense RNA hunts for a matching sequence on the mRNA (or sense RNA) encoding for some protein. When the antisense RNA binds to the sense RNA, the expression of the gene that encoded the sense RNA (or mRNA) is blocked. Therefore, antisense RNAs seem to be very potent blockers of gene expression. (mRNA, messenger RNA.) **C:** Riboswitch *RNA* genes. The riboswitch RNA folds into a complex three-dimensional shape, where one portion recognizes a target molecule and the other portion contains a protein-coding RNA sequence. When the riboswitch RNA binds to the target molecule, the "switch" is turned on and the protein-coding RNA sequence is translated into a protein product. (3D, three dimensional.)

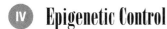 Epigenetic Control

A. CHEMICAL MODIFICATION OF DNA.

   1. DNA can be chemically modified by **methylation of cytosine nucleotides** using **methylating enzymes.** An increased methylation of a DNA segment will make that DNA segment less likely to be transcribed into RNA, and hence any genes in that DNA segment will be silenced (i.e., ↑**methylation of DNA = silenced genes**). The DNA nucleotide sequence is not altered by these modifications.

   2. DNA methylation plays a crucial role in the epigenetic phenomenon called *genomic imprinting*. Genomic imprinting is the differential expression of alleles depending on whether the allele is on the paternal chromosome or the maternal chromosome.

   3. When a gene is imprinted, only the allele on the paternal chromosome is expressed, while the allele on the maternal chromosome is silenced (or vice versa).

   4. During male and female gametogenesis, male and female chromosomes acquire some sort of **imprint** that signals the difference between paternal and maternal alleles. However, all of the mechanisms involved in the imprinting process are not well elucidated.

B. CHEMICAL MODIFICATION OF HISTONES. Histone proteins can be chemically modified by **acetylation, methylation, phosphorylation,** or the **addition of ubiquitin** (sometimes called *epigenetic marks* or *epigenetic tags*). An increased acetylation of histone proteins will make a DNA segment more likely to be transcribed into RNA, and hence any genes in that DNA segment will be expressed (i.e., ↑**acetylation of histones = expressed genes**). The mechanism that determines the location and combination of epigenetic tags is unknown.

Ⓥ Noncoding DNA

A. SATELLITE DNA. Satellite DNA is composed of very large-sized blocks (100 kb → several Mb) of **tandemly repeated noncoding DNA.**

B. MINISATELLITE DNA. Minisatellite DNA is composed of moderately sized blocks (0.1 kb → 20.0 kb) of **tandemly repeated noncoding DNA.**

C. MICROSATELLITE DNA (Simple Sequence Repeat [SSR]). Microsatellite DNA is composed of small-sized blocks (<100 bp) of **tandemly repeated noncoding DNA.** Microsatellite DNA consists of a <10 bp repeat unit and is found dispersed throughout all of the chromosomes.

D. TRANSPOSONS (Transposable Elements; "Jumping Genes"). Transposons are composed of **interspersed repetitive noncoding DNA** that make up an incredible 45% of the human nuclear genome. Transposons are mobile DNA sequences that jump from one place in the genome to another (called *transposition*).

   1. Types of transposons.

   a. **Short interspersed nuclear elements (SINEs).** SINEs are classified into three families: **Alu, MIR,** and **MIR3.** The **Alu repeat** (280 bp) is a SINE that is the **most abundant sequence in the human genome.**

b. **Long interspersed nuclear elements (LINEs).** LINEs are classified into three families: **LINE1**, **LINE 2**, and **LINE 3**. LINE 1 ($\approx$6.1 kb) is the **most important human transposon** in that it is still actively transposing (jumping) and may disrupt important functioning genes.

c. **Long terminal repeat (LTR) transposons.** LTR transposons are classified into two families: **ERV** and **MaLR**.

d. **DNA transposons.** DNA transposons are classified into two families: **MER-1** (**Charlie**) and **MER-2** (**Tigger**). Most DNA transposons in humans are no longer active (i.e., they do not jump) and therefore are considered *transposon fossils.*

2. **Mechanism of transposition (Figure 1-3A, B).** Transposable elements jump either as double-stranded DNA using **conservative transposition** (a "cut-and-paste" method) or through a RNA intermediate using **retrotransposition.**

a. **Conservative transposition.** In conservative transposition, the transposon jumps as double-stranded DNA. **Transposase** (a recombination enzyme similar to an integrase) cuts the transposable element at a site marked by **inverted repeat DNA sequences** ($\approx$20 bp long). Transposase is encoded in the DNA of the transposable element. The transposon is inserted at a new location, perhaps on another chromosome. This mechanism is similar to the mechanism that a **DNA virus** uses in its life cycle to transform host DNA.

b. **Retrotransposition.** In retrotransposition, the transposon jumps through a RNA intermediate. The transposon undergoes transcription, which produces a RNA copy that encodes a reverse transcriptase enzyme. **Reverse transcriptase** makes a double-stranded DNA copy of the transposon from the RNA copy. The transposon is inserted at a new location using the enzyme **integrase**. This mechanism is similar to the mechanism that a **RNA virus (retrovirus)** uses in its life cycle to transform host DNA.

3. **Transposons and genetic variability (Figure 1-3C–F).** The main effect of transposons is to affect the genetic variability of the organism. Transposons can do this in several ways:

a. **Mutation at the former site of the transposon.** After the transposon is cut out of its site in the host chromosome by transposase, the host DNA must undergo DNA repair. A mutation may arise at the repair site.

b. **Level of gene expression.** If the transposon moves to the target DNA near an active gene, the transposon may affect the level of expression of that gene. While most of these changes in the level of gene expression would be detrimental to the organism, some of the changes over time might be beneficial and then spread through the population.

c. **Gene inactivation.** If the transposon moves to the target DNA in the middle of a gene sequence, the gene will be mutated and may be inactivated.

d. **Gene transfer.** If two transposons happen to be close to one another, the transposition mechanism may cut the ends of two different transposons. This will move the DNA between the two transposons to a new location. If that DNA contains a gene (or an exon sequence), then the gene will be transferred to a new location. This mechanism is especially important in **development of antibiotic resistance** in bacteria. Transposons in bacterial DNA can move to bacteriophage DNA, which can then spread to other bacteria. If the bacterial DNA between the two transposons contains the gene for tetracycline resistance, then other bacteria will become tetracycline resistant.

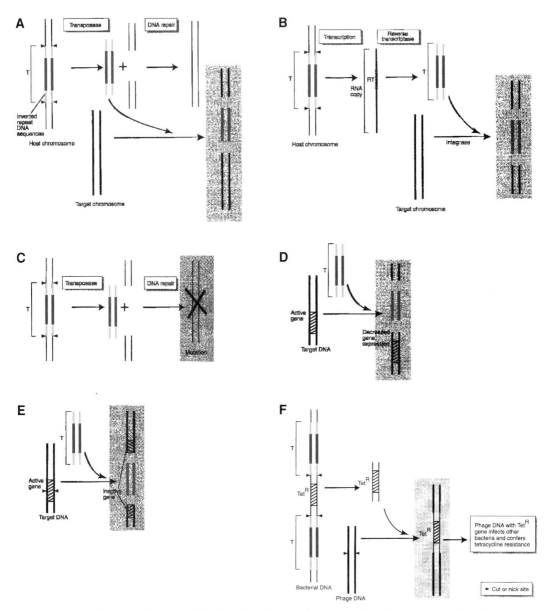

● **Figure 1-3 Mechanisms of transposition (A, B). A:** Conservative transposition. **B:** Retrotransposition. **Transposons and genetic variability (C–F). C:** Mutation at the former site of the transposon. **D:** Level of gene expression. **E:** Gene inactivation. **F:** Gene transfer. (T, transposon; RT, RNA code for reverse transcriptase (^): cut sites Tet^R: gene for tetracycline resistance.)

Chapter 2

DNA Packaging

Ⅰ **The Biochemistry of Nucleic Acids (Figure 2-1).** A **nucleoside** consists of a nitrogenous base and a sugar. A **nucleotide** consists of a nitrogenous base, a sugar, and a phosphate group. DNA and RNA consist of a chain of nucleotides that are composed of the following components:

A. NITROGENOUS BASES.
　1. **Purines.**
　　a. Adenine (A).
　　b. Guanine (G).
　2. **Pyrimidines.**
　　a. Cytosine (C).
　　b. Thymine (T).
　　c. Uracil (U), which is found in RNA.
　3. **Base pairing.** Adenine pairs with thymine or uracil (**A-T or A-U**). Cytosine pairs with guanine (**C-G**).

B. SUGARS.
　1. Deoxyribose, which is found in DNA.
　2. Ribose, which is found in RNA.

C. PHOSPHATE (PO_4^{3-}).

Ⅱ **Levels of DNA Packaging (Figure 2-2)**

A. DOUBLE HELIX DNA.
　1. The DNA molecule is two complementary polynucleotide chains (or DNA strands) arranged as a double helix that are held together by **hydrogen bonding** between laterally opposed base pairs (bp).
　2. DNA can adopt different helical structures that include **A-DNA** and **B-DNA**, which are right-handed helices with 11 bp and 10 bp per turn, respectively; and **Z-DNA**, which is a left-handed helix with 12 bp per turn. In humans, most of the DNA is in the B-DNA form under physiologic conditions.

B. NUCLEOSOME.
　1. The most fundamental unit of packaging of DNA is the nucleosome. A nucleosome consists of a histone protein octamer (two each of **H2A, H2B, H3, and H4 histone proteins**), around which 146 bp of DNA is coiled in 1.75 turns.
　2. The nucleosomes are connected by spacer DNA, which results in a 10-nm-diameter fiber that resembles a "beads on a string" appearance by electron microscopy.

3. Histones are small proteins containing a high proportion of **lysine** and **arginine** that impart a positive charge to the proteins, which enhances its binding to negatively charged DNA in A-T-rich regions.

4. **Histone acetylation** of lysine by **histone acetyltransferases (HATs)** reduces the affinity between histones and DNA.

5. An increased acetylation of histone proteins will make a DNA segment more likely to be transcribed into RNA; hence, any genes in that DNA segment will be expressed (i.e., ↑acetylation of histones = expressed genes).

C. 30-nm CHROMATIN FIBER.

1. The 10-nm nucleosome fiber is joined by **H1 histone protein** to form a **30-nm chromatin fiber.**

2. During the interphase of mitosis, chromosomes exist as 30-nm chromatin fibers organized as **extended chromatin.** When the general term *chromatin* is used, it refers specifically to the 30-nm chromatin fiber organized as extended chromatin.

3. The extended chromatin can also form **secondary loops.**

4. During metaphase of mitosis, chromatin undergoes **compaction.**

Ⅲ Centromere

A. A centromere is a specialized nucleotide DNA sequence that binds to the mitotic spindle during cell division.

B. A major component of centromeric DNA is **α-satellite DNA,** which consists of a 171-bp repeat unit along with **β-satellite DNA** (a 68-bp repeat unit) and **satellite 1 DNA** (a 25–48-bp repeat unit).

C. A centromere is associated with a number of centromeric proteins that include **CENP-A, CENP-B** (which binds to a 17-bp sequence in α-satellite DNA), **CENP-C,** and **CENP-G.**

D. Chromosomes have a single centromere that is observed microscopically as a **primary constriction,** which is the region where sister chromatids are joined.

E. During prometaphase, a pair of protein complexes called *kinetochores* forms at the centromere, and one kinetochore is attached to each sister chromatid.

F. Microtubules produced the by **centrosome** of the cell attach to the kinetochore (called *kinetochore microtubules*) and pull the two sister chromatids toward opposite poles of the mitotic cell.

Ⅳ Heterochromatin and Euchromatin

A. **Heterochromatin** is condensed chromatin and is **transcriptionally inactive.** In electron micrographs, heterochromatin is electron dense (i.e., very black). An example of heterochromatin is the **Barr body** that can be seen in interphase cells from females, which is the inactive X chromosome. Heterochromatin comprises ≈10% of the total chromatin.

1. **Constitutive heterochromatin** is always condensed (i.e., transcriptionally inactive) and consists of repetitive DNA found near the centromere and other regions.

2. **Facultative heterochromatin** can be either condensed (i.e., transcriptionally inactive) or dispersed (i.e., transcriptionally active). An example of facultative heterochromatin is the **XY body,** which forms when both the X and Y chromosome are inactivated for ≈15 days during male meiosis and when the X chromosome is inactivated in females.

B. **Euchromatin** is dispersed chromatin and comprises ≈90% of the total chromatin. Of this 90%, 10% is transcriptionally active and 80% is transcriptionally inactive. When chromatin is transcriptionally active, there is weak binding to the H1 histone protein and **acetylation** of the H2A, H2B, H3, and H4 histone proteins.

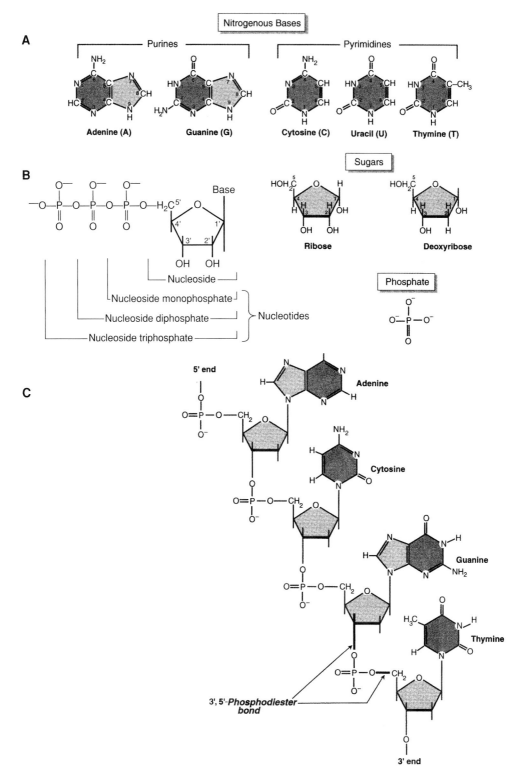

● **Figure 2-1 Biochemistry of DNA. A:** Structure of the biochemical components of DNA and RNA (purines, pyrimidines, sugars, and phosphate). **B:** Diagram depicting the chemical structure of the various components of DNA. **C:** Diagram of a DNA polynucleotide chain. The biochemical components (purines, pyrimidines, sugar, and phosphate) form a polynucleotide chain through a 3′,5′-phosphodiester bond.

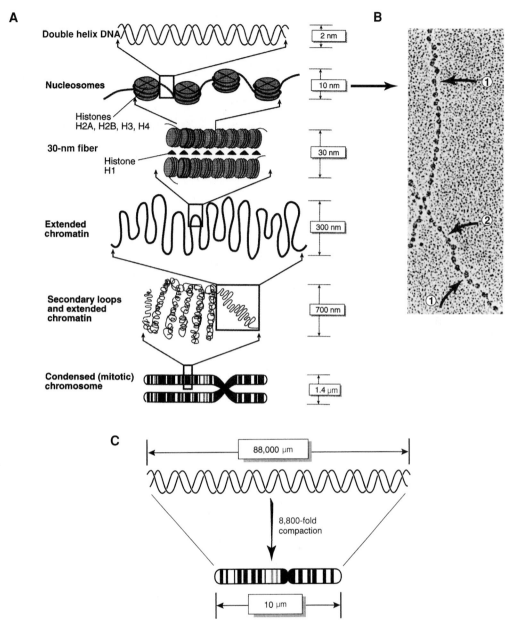

A

Double helix DNA [2 nm]

Nucleosomes [10 nm]

Histones
H2A, H2B, H3, H4

30-nm fiber [30 nm]

Histone
H1

Extended
chromatin [300 nm]

Secondary loops
and extended
chromatin [700 nm]

Condensed (mitotic)
chromosome [1.4 µm]

B

① ② ①

C

[88,000 µm]

8,800-fold
compaction

[10 µm]

● **Figure 2-2 DNA packaging. A:** Diagram depicting the various levels of packaging of double helix DNA found within a metaphase chromosome. Double helix DNA is wound around a histone octamer of H2A, H2B, H3, and H4 to form a **nucleosome.** Nucleosomes are pulled together by histone H1 to form a 30-nm-diameter fiber. The 30-nm fiber exists either as **extended chromatin** or as **secondary loops** within a condensed metaphase chromosome. **B:** Electron micrograph of DNA isolated and subjected to treatments that unfold DNA to a nucleosome. The **"beads on a string"** appearance is the basic unit of chromatin packaging, called a *nucleosome.* The globular structure ("bead") (*arrow 1*) is a histone octamer. The linear structure ("string") (*arrow 2*) is DNA. **C:** Compaction of DNA in a chromosome. The double helix DNA of a chromosome is shown unraveled and stretched out, measuring 88,000 µm in length. During the metaphase of mitosis, chromatin can become highly compacted. For example, human chromosome 1 contains about 260,000,000 bp. The distance between each base pair is 0.34 nm. Therefore, the physical length of the DNA comprising chromosome 1 is 88,000,000 nm or 88,000 µm (260,000,000 × 0.34 nm = 88,000,000 nm). During the metaphase, all of the chromosomes condense such that the physical length of chromosome 1 is about 10 µm. Consequently, the 88,000 µm of DNA comprising chromosome 1 is reduced to 10 µm, resulting in an 8,800-fold compaction.

Chapter 3

Protein Synthesis

I. General Features

A. The flow of genetic information in a cell is almost exclusively in one direction: DNA→RNA→protein and follows a **colinearity principle** in that a *linear sequence* of nucleotides in DNA is decoded to give a *linear sequence* of nucleotides in RNA that is decoded to give a *linear sequence* of amino acids in a protein.

B. This flow involves three main successive steps, including **transcription, processing the RNA transcript**, and **translation**.

II. Transcription

A. TRANSCRIPTION IN GENERAL.

1. Transcription is the mechanism by which the cell copies **DNA into RNA** and occurs in the **nucleus**. During transcription, the double helix DNA is unwound, and the **DNA template strand** forms transient **RNA-DNA hybrid** with the growing RNA transcript. The other DNA strand is called the *DNA nontemplate strand.*

2. DNA sequences that flank the gene sequence at the 5′ end of the template strand are called *upstream sequences*. DNA sequences that flank the gene sequence at the 3′ end of the template strand are called *downstream sequences*.

3. Transcription is carried out by **DNA-directed RNA polymerase** that copies a DNA template strand in the **3′→5′ direction**, which in turn produces a RNA transcript in the **5′→3′ direction**. There are three RNA polymerases, as indicated in Table 3-1.

TABLE 3-1	RNA POLYMERASE FUNCTIONS
Polymerase	**Function**
RNA polymerase I	Produces 45S rRNA
RNA polymerase II	Produces a RNA transcript that is further processed into mRNA (used in protein synthesis)
RNA polymerase III	Produces 5S rRNA, tRNA, snRNAs, snoRNA, and miRNA

rRNA, ribosomal RNA; mRNA, messenger RNA; tRNA, transfer RNA; snRNA, small nuclear RNA; snoRNA, small nucleolar RNA; miRNA, microRNA.

B. TRANSCRIPTION IN PROTEIN SYNTHESIS

1. During protein synthesis, RNA polymerase II produces a RNA transcript by a complex process that involves a number of **general transcription factors** called *transcription factors for RNA polymerase II* (**TFIIs**) that are further processed into messenger RNA (mRNA).

2. **TFIID** binds to the **TATA box**, which then allows the adjacent binding of **TFIIB**. The next step involves **TFIIA, TFIIE, TFIIF,** TFIIH, and **RNA polymerase II** engaged to the promoter, forming a **transcription initiation (TI) complex**.
3. The TI complex must gain access to the DNA template strand at the transcription start site, which is accomplished by a **DNA helicase**.
4. The TI complex will produce only a **basal level of transcription** or **constitutive expression**. Other factors called *cis-acting DNA sequences* and *trans-acting proteins* are necessary for high levels of expression.

III Processing the RNA Transcript into mRNA (Figure 3-1). A cell involved in protein synthesis will use RNA polymerase II to transcribe a protein-coding gene into a **RNA transcript** that must be further processed into mRNA. This processing involves the following:

A. RNA CAPPING
1. RNA capping is the addition of a **7-methylguanosine** to the first nucleotide at the 5′ **end** of the RNA transcript.
2. RNA capping functions are to protect the RNA transcript from exonuclease attack, to facilitate transport from the nucleus to the cytoplasm, to facilitate RNA splicing, and to attach the mRNA to the 40S subunit of the ribosome.

B. RNA POLYADENYLATION
1. RNA polyadenylation is the addition of a **poly-A tail** (about 200 repeated AMPs) to the 3′ **end** of the RNA transcript.
2. The **AAUAAA sequence** is a **polyadenylation signal sequence** that signals the 3′ cleavage of the RNA transcript. After 3′ cleavage, polyadenylation occurs.
3. RNA polyadenylation functions are to protect against degradation, to facilitate transport from the nucleus to the cytoplasm, and to enhance recognition of the mRNA by the ribosomes.

C. RNA SPLICING
1. RNA splicing is a process whereby all **introns (noncoding regions; intervening sequences)** are removed from the RNA transcript, and all **exons (coding regions; expression sequences)** are joined together within the RNA transcript.
2. RNA splicing requires that the intron/exon boundaries (or **splice junctions**) be recognized. In most cases, introns start with a GT (GU at the RNA level) sequence and end with a AG sequence (called the *GT-AG rule*).
3. RNA splicing is carried out by a large RNA-protein complex called the *spliceosome*, which consists of **five types of small nuclear RNA (snRNA)** (i.e., **U1 snRNA, U2 snRNA, U4 snRNA, U5 snRNA, and U6 snRNA**) and more than **50 different proteins**. Each snRNA is complexed to specific proteins to form **small ribonucleoprotein particles (snRNPs)**.
4. The RNA portion of the snRNPs hybridizes to a nucleotide sequence that marks the intron site (GT-AG rule), whereas the protein portion cuts out the intron and rejoins the RNA transcript.
5. This produces mRNA that can leave the nucleus and be translated in the cytoplasm.

Ⓘ Translation (Figure 3-2)

A. Translation is the mechanism by which only the centrally located nucleotide **sequence of mRNA** is translated into the **amino acid sequence of a protein** and occurs in the **cytoplasm.**

B. The end or flanking sequences of the mRNA (called the **5′ and 3′ untranslated regions; 5′UTR** and **3′UTR**) are not translated.

C. Translation decodes a set of **three** nucleotides (called a *codon*) into **one** amino acid (e.g., GCA codes for alanine, UAC codes for tyrosine, etc.). The code is said to be **redundant,** which means that more than one codon specifies a particular amino acid (e.g., GCA, GCC, GCG, and GCU all specify alanine, and UAC and UAU both specify tyrosine).

D. Translation uses **transfer RNA (tRNA)**, which has two important binding sites. The first site of tRNA, called the *anticodon*, binds to the complementary codon on the mRNA and demonstrates **tRNA wobble,** whereby the normal A-U and G-C pairing is required only in the first two base positions of the codon, but variability or wobble occurs at the third position. The second site of tRNA is the **amino acid–binding site** on the acceptor arm, which covalently binds the amino acid to the 3′ end of tRNA.

E. Translation uses the enzyme **aminoacyl-tRNA synthetase,** which links an amino acid to tRNA. **tRNA charging** refers to the fact that the amino acid–tRNA bond contains the energy for the formation of the peptide bond between amino acids. There is a specific aminoacyl-tRNA synthetase for each amino acid. Since there are 20 different amino acids, there are 20 different aminoacyl-tRNA synthetase enzymes.

F. Translation uses the enzyme **peptidyl transferase,** which participates in forming the peptide bond between amino acids of the growing protein.

G. Translation requires the use of ribosomes, which are large RNA-protein complexes that consist of a **40S subunit** (consisting of 18S rRNA and ≈30 ribosomal proteins) and a **60S subunit** (consisting of 5S rRNA, 5.8 rRNA, 28S rRNA, and ~50 ribosomal proteins). The ribosome moves along the mRNA in a **5′→3′ direction** such that the **NH2-terminal end** of a protein is synthesized **first** and the **COOH-terminal end** of a protein is synthesized **last.**

H. Translation begins with the start **codon AUG** that codes for **methionine** (the optimal initiation codon recognition sequence is **GCACCAUGG**) so that all newly synthesized proteins have methionine as their first (or NH2-terminal) amino acid, which is usually removed later by a protease.

I. Translation terminates at the **stop codon (UAA, UAG, UGA).** The stop codon binds **release factors** that cause the protein to be released from the ribosome into the cytoplasm.

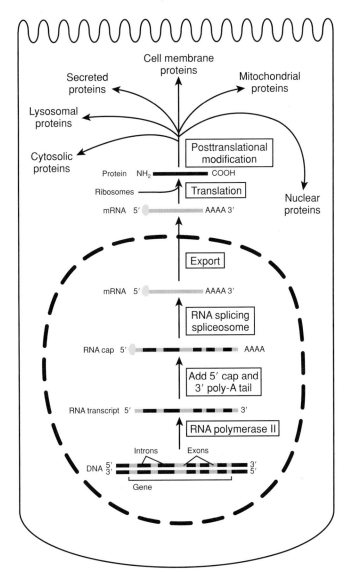

● **Figure 3-1 Transcription and processing of RNA into mRNA.** All eucaryotic genes contain noncoding regions (introns) separated by coding regions (exons). During transcription, RNA polymerase II transcribes both intron and exon sequences into a RNA transcript. A 5′ cap and a 3′ poly-A tail are added. The introns are spliced out of the RNA transcript by a spliceosome so that all the exons are joined in sequence. The mRNA with the 5′ cap and 3′ poly-A tail is then able to exit the nucleus through the nuclear pore complex into the cytoplasm for subsequent translation into protein. Proteins then undergo posttranslational modifications and are directed to various regions of the cell.

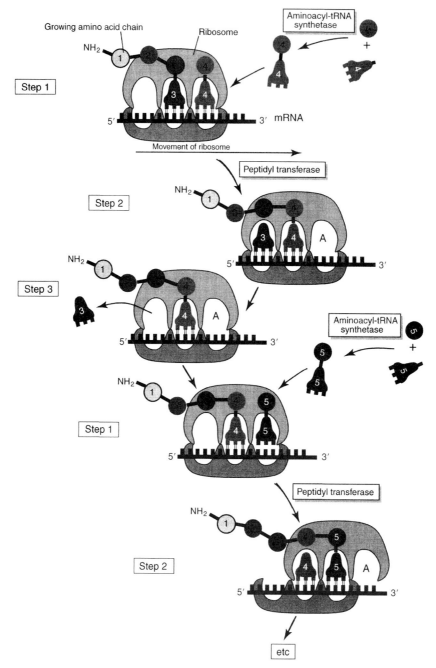

● **Figure 3-2 Translation.** This diagram joins the process of translation at a point where three amino acids have already been linked together (amino acids 1, 2, and 3). The process of translation is basically a three-step process that is repeated over and over during the synthesis of a protein. The enzyme aminoacyl-tRNA synthetase links a specific amino acid with its specific tRNA. In step 1, the tRNA and amino acid complex 4 binds to the A site on the ribosome. Note that the direction of movement of the ribosome along the mRNA is in a 5'→3' direction. In step 2, the enzyme peptidyl transferase forms a peptide bond between amino acid 3 and amino acid 4, and the small subunit of the ribosome reconfigures so that the A site is vacant. In step 3, the used tRNA 3 is ejected, and the ribosome is ready for tRNA and amino acid complex 5.

Chapter 4

Chromosome Replication

I. General Features

A. Chromosome replication occurs during the **S phase** of the cell cycle and involves both DNA synthesis and histone synthesis to form chromatin.

B. The timing of replication is related to the chromatin structure. An **inactive gene** packaged as **heterochromatin** is replicated **late in the S phase** (e.g., in a female mammalian cell, the inactive X chromosome called the *Barr body* is packaged as heterochromatin and is replicated late in the S phase).

C. An **active gene** packaged as **euchromatin** is replicated early in the S phase (e.g., in the pancreatic beta cell, the insulin gene will be replicated early in the S phase. However, in other cell types (e.g., hepatocytes) where the insulin gene is inactive, it will be replicated late in the S phase.

D. DNA polymerases absolutely require the **3′-OH end** of a base-paired primer strand as a substrate for strand extension. Therefore, a **RNA primer** (synthesized by a **primase**) is required to provide the free 3′-OH group needed to start DNA synthesis.

E. DNA polymerases copy a DNA template in the **3′→5′ direction**, which produces a new DNA strand in the **5′→3′ direction**.

F. **Deoxyribonucleoside 5′-triphosphates (dATP, dTTP, dGTP, dCTP)** pair with the corresponding base (A-T, G-C) on the template strand and form a **3′,5′-phosphodiester bond** with the **3′-OH group on the deoxyribose sugar**, which releases a **pyrophosphate**.

G. Replication is described as **semiconservative**, which means that a molecule of double helix DNA contains one intact parental DNA strand and one newly synthesized DNA strand.

II. The Replication Process (Figure 4-1)

A. The process starts when **topoisomerase** nicks (or breaks) a single strand of DNA, which causes DNA unwinding.

B. Chromosome replication begins at specific nucleotide sequences located throughout the chromosome called *replication origins*. Eukaryotic DNA contains **multiple replication origins** to ensure rapid DNA synthesis. Normally, the S phase of the mammalian cell cycle is **8 hours**.

C. **DNA** helicase recognizes the replication origin and opens up the double helix at that site, forming a **replication bubble** with a **replication fork** at each end. The stability of the replication fork is maintained by **single-stranded binding proteins**.

D. A replication fork contains the following elements:
1. A **leading strand** that is synthesized continuously by **DNA polymerase delta (δ)**.
2. A **lagging strand** that is synthesized discontinuously by **DNA polymerase alpha (α)**. **DNA primase** synthesizes short RNA primers along the lagging strand. DNA polymerase α uses the RNA primer to synthesize DNA fragments called *Okazaki fragments*. Okazaki fragments end when they run into a downstream RNA primer. To form a continuous DNA strand from the Okazaki fragments, a **DNA repair enzyme** removes the RNA primers and replaces it with DNA. **DNA ligase** subsequently joins the all the DNA fragments together.

E. The antineoplastic drugs **camptothecins** (e.g., **irinotecan, topotecan**), **anthracyclines** (e.g., **doxorubicin**), **epipodophyllotoxins** (e.g., **etoposide VP-16, teniposide VM-26**), and **amsacrine** are topoisomerase inhibitors.

F. The antimicrobial drugs **quinolones** (e.g., **ciprofloxacin, ofloxacin, levofloxacin, fluoroquinolones**) are also topoisomerase inhibitors.

Ⅲ The Telomere

A. The human telomere is a 3–20 kb repeating nucleotide sequence (**TTAGGG**) located at the end of a chromosome. The 3–20 kb (TTAGGG)$_n$ array is preceded by 100–300 kb of telomere-associated repeats before any unique sequence is found.

B. The telomere allows replication of linear DNA to its full length. Since DNA polymerases <u>CANNOT</u> synthesize in the 3'→5' direction or start synthesis de novo, removal of the RNA primers will always leave the 5' end of the lagging strand shorter than the leading strand. If the 5' end of the lagging strand is not lengthened, a chromosome would become progressively shorter as the cell goes through a number of cell divisions.

C. Telomerase is <u>NOT</u> utilized by a majority of **normal somatic cells**, so chromosomes normally become successively shorter after each replication, which contributes to the finite life span of the cell.

D. Telomerase is utilized by **stems cells** and **neoplastic cells**, so chromosomes remain perpetually long. Telomerase may play a clinical role in **aging** and **cancer**.

E. This problem is solved by a special **RNA-directed DNA polymerase or reverse transcriptase** called *telomerase* (which has a RNA and protein component). The RNA component of telomerase carries a **CCCUAA** sequence (antisense sequence of the TTAGGG telomere), recognizes the TTAGGG sequence on the leading strand, and adds many repeats of TTAGGG to the leading strand.

F. After the repeats of TTAGGG are added to the leading strand, **DNA polymerase α** uses the TTAGGG repeats as a template to synthesize the complementary repeats on the lagging strand. Thus, the lagging strand is lengthened. **DNA ligase** joins the repeats to the lagging strand, and a **nuclease** cleaves the ends to form double helix DNA with flush ends.

IV Types of DNA Damage and DNA Repair

A. Chromosomal breakage refers to breaks in chromosomes due to sunlight (or ultraviolet) irradiation, ionizing irradiation, DNA cross-linking agents, or DNA damaging agents. These insults may cause **depurination of DNA, deamination of cytosine to uracil,** or **pyrimidine dimerization** that must be repaired by DNA repair enzymes.

B. DNA repair involves **DNA excision** of the damaged site, **DNA synthesis** of the correct sequence, and **DNA ligation.** Some types of DNA repair use enzymes that do not require DNA excision.

C. The normal response to DNA damage is to stall the cell in the G_1 **phase** of the cell cycle until the damage is repaired.

D. The system that detects and signals DNA damage is a multiprotein complex called *BRCA1-associated genome surveillance complex* (**BASC**). (Some of the components of BASC include **ataxia telangiectasia mutated (ATM) protein, nibrin, BRCA1 protein,** and **BRCA2 protein**).

E. The clinical importance of DNA repair enzymes is illustrated by some rare inherited diseases that involve genetic defects in DNA repair enzymes such as xeroderma pigmentosa (XP), ataxia-telangiectasia, Fanconi anemia, Bloom syndrome, and hereditary nonpolyposis colorectal cancer.

F. Types of DNA damage include the following:
1. **Depurination.** About 5,000 purines (A's or G's) per day are lost from DNA of each human cell when the N-glycosyl bond between the purine and deoxyribose sugar-phosphate is broken. This is the most frequent type of lesion and leaves the deoxyribose sugar-phosphate with a missing purine base.
2. **Deamination of cytosine to uracil.** About 100 cytosines (C) per day are spontaneously deaminated to uracil (U). If the U is not corrected back to a C, then on replication, instead of the occurrence of a correct C-G base pairing, a U-A base pairing will occur.
3. **Pyrimidine dimerization.** Sunlight (UV radiation) can cause covalent linkage of adjacent pyrimidines, forming, for example, **thymine dimers.**

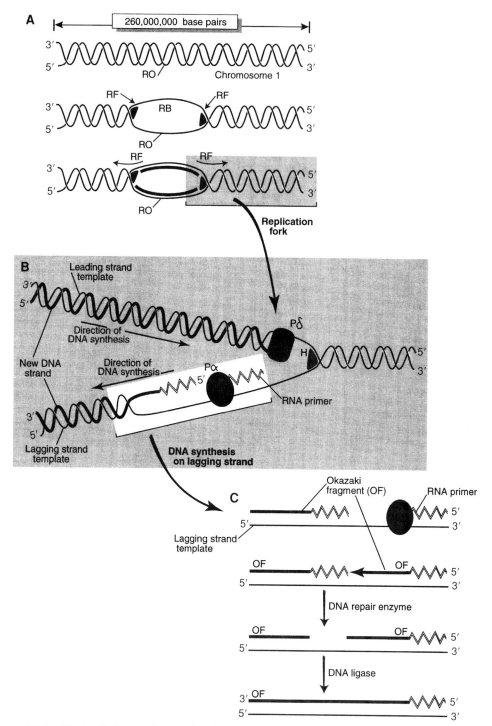

● **Figure 4-1 Replication fork. A:** A diagram of double helix DNA (*Chromosome 1*) at a replication origin (*RO*) site. DNA helicase will bind at the replication origin and unwind the double helix into two DNA strands. This site is called a *replication bubble* (*RB*). At both ends of a replication bubble, a replication fork (*RF*) forms. DNA synthesis occurs in a bidirectional manner from each replication fork (*arrows*). **B:** Enlarged view of a replication fork at one end of the replication bubble. The leading strand serves as a template for continuous DNA synthesis in the 5'→3' direction using DNA polymerase δ (*Pδ*). The lagging strand serves as a template for discontinuous DNA synthesis in the 5'→3' direction using DNA polymerase α (*Pα*). Note that DNA synthesis on the leading and lagging strands is in the 5'→3' direction but physically are running in opposite directions. **C:** DNA synthesis on the lagging strand proceeds differently from that on the leading strand. DNA primase synthesizes RNA primers. DNA polymerase α uses these RNA primers to synthesize DNA fragments called *Okazaki fragments* (*OF*). Okazaki fragments end when they run into a downstream RNA primer. Subsequently, DNA repair enzymes remove the RNA primers and replace it with DNA. Finally, DNA ligase joins all of the Okazaki fragments together.

Chapter 5

Mendelian Inheritance

I Autosomal Dominant Inheritance (Figure 5-1A, B; Table 5-1)

A. INTRODUCTION. In autosomal dominant inheritance, the disease is caused by a mutation in a single gene and is observed **with equal probability in both males and females** who are **heterozygous** for the mutant gene. Homozygotes for autosomal dominant diseases rarely occur, and the double dominant condition usually is embryonic lethal. The characteristic family pedigree is **vertical**, in that the disease is passed from one generation to the next. Recurrence risk is 50% for an affected parent with each pregnancy.

B. NEW MUTATIONS. In autosomal dominant diseases, new mutations are relatively common. In these cases, there will be an affected child with no family history of the disease. There is a low recurrence risk (1%–2%) due to the possibility of germ line mosaicism. Germ line mosaicism is the presence of more than one cell line in the gametes in an otherwise normal parent and is the result of a mutation during the embryonic development of that parent. There is an increased risk for a new dominant mutation in fathers over 50 years of age.

C. REDUCED PENETRANCE. In a reduced penetrance, many individuals have the disease mutation but do not develop disease symptoms. However, they can still transmit the disease mutation and have affected offspring. *Example:* Breast cancer, whereby many women have mutations in the *BRCA1* gene and *BRCA2* genes but do not develop the disease. However, some women have mutations in the *BRCA1* gene and *BRCA2* genes and do develop breast cancer.

D. VARIABLE EXPRESSIVITY. In variable expressivity, the severity of the disease can vary greatly between individuals. Some people may have such mild disease that they do not know they have it until a severely affected child is born. *Example:* Marfan syndrome, whereby a parent is tall and has long fingers, but one of his children is tall, has long fingers, and has serious cardiovascular defects.

E. PLEIOTROPY. Pleiotropy refers to a situation when a disease has multiple effects on the body. *Example:* Marfan syndrome, whereby the eye, skeleton, and cardiovascular system may be affected.

F. LOCUS HETEROGENEITY. In locus heterogeneity, genes at more than one locus may cause the disease. *Example:* Osteogenesis imperfecta, whereby collagen a-1(I) chain protein and collagen a-2(I) chain protein are encoded by the *COL1A1* gene on chromosome 17q21.3-q22 and *COL1A2* gene on chromosome 7q22.1, respectively (i.e., two separate genes located on different chromosomes). A mutation in either gene will cause osteogenesis imperfecta.

G. EXAMPLES OF AUTOSOMAL DOMINANT DISORDERS.

1. Huntington disease (HD).

a. HD is an autosomal dominant genetic disorder caused by a 36 → 100 + unstable repeat sequence of (CAG)n located in the *HD* gene on **chromosome 4p16.3** for the **huntingtin** protein, which is a widely expressed cytoplasmic protein present in neurons within the striatum, cerebral cortex, and cerebellum, although its precise function is unknown.

b. Since CAG codes for the amino acid glutamine, a long tract of glutamines (a polyglutamine tract) will be inserted into the huntingtin protein and cause protein aggregates to form within certain cells (such as implicated in other neurodegenerative disorders).

c. **Clinical features include**: age of onset is 35–44 years of age, mean survival time is 15–18 years after onset, a movement jerkiness that is most apparent at movement termination, chorea (dancelike movements), memory deficits, affective disturbances, personality changes, dementia, diffuse and marked atrophy of the neostriatum due to cell death of cholinergic neurons and GABA-ergic neurons within the striatum (caudate nucleus and putamen) and a relative increase in dopaminergic neuron activity, and neuronal intranuclear aggregates. The disease is protracted and invariably fatal. In HD, homozygotes are not more severely affected by the disease than heterozygotes, which is an exception in autosomal dominant disorders.

2. Neurofibromatosis type 1 (von Recklinghausen disease; see Chapter 7).

3. Marfan syndrome (see Chapter 13).

4. Osteogenesis imperfecta (see Chapter 13).

5. Achondroplasia (see Chapter 13).

Ⅱ Autosomal Recessive Inheritance (Figure 5-1C; Table 5-1)

A. INTRODUCTION.
In autosomal recessive inheritance, the disease is observed **with equal probability in both males and females** who are **homozygous** for the mutant gene. The characteristic pedigree is **horizontal**, in that affected individuals tend to be limited to a single sibship and the disease is not found in multiple generations. The parents of a proband are obligate heterozygotes whereby each parent carries one mutant allele and is asymptomatic. The risk to the siblings of the proband is a 25% chance of having the disease (aa), a 50% chance of being a normal heterozygote carrier (Aa), and a 25% chance of being a normal homozygous individual (AA). Consanguinity increases the risk for autosomal recessive diseases in the children.

B. EXAMPLES OF AUTOSOMAL RECESSIVE DISORDERS.

1. Cystic fibrosis (CF).

a. CF is an autosomal recessive genetic disorder caused by >1,000 mutations in the *CFTR* gene on **chromosome 7q31.2** for the **c**ystic **f**ibrosis **t**ransmembrane conductance **r**egulator, which functions as a chloride ion (Cl^-) channel.

b. CF is most commonly (≈70% of cases in the North American population) caused by a **three base deletion** that codes for the amino acid **phenylalanine at position #508** (delta F508) such that phenylalanine is missing from CFTR. However, there are a large number of deletions that can cause CF, and parents of an affected child can carry different deletions of CFTR. These mutations result in absent/near absent CFTR synthesis, a block in CFTR regulation, or a destruction of Cl^- transport.

c.   **Clinical features include**: production of abnormally thick mucus by epithelial cells lining the respiratory tract resulting in obstruction of pulmonary airways, recurrent respiratory bacterial infections, and end-stage lung disease; pancreatic insufficiency with malabsorption; acute salt depletion and chronic metabolic alkalosis; males are almost always sterile due to the obstruction or absence of the vas deferens; and whites are the most commonly affected ethnic group, with CF occurring in 1 in 2,500 live births.

2.   Sickle cell disease (SCD).

a.   SCD is an autosomal recessive genetic disorder caused by a mutation in the *HBB* **gene** on **chromosome 11p15.5** for the **hemoglobin β-subunit** that is involved in oxygen transport by red blood cells.

b.   SCD is most commonly caused by a missense mutation that results in a **normal glutamic acid→valine** substitution at position 6 (E6V) and the presence of **hemoglobin S** (Hb S; called *sickle cell disease*).

c.   In homozygotes, this mutation alters the structure of the hemoglobin molecule in such a way that erythrocytes become sickle-shaped under low oxygen conditions and cannot pass through capillaries, leading to blockages of these vessels.

d.   Individuals who are heterozygous for the mutant gene, and thus carriers of "sickle cell trait," are normally not affected but may experience a painful crisis under very low oxygen pressure. However, heterozygotes may have a resistance to malaria. The mutation is relatively common in blacks, with 1 in 12 individuals being carriers.

e.   SCD may also be caused by coinheritance of the E6V mutation along with another missense mutation that results in a **normal glutamic acid→lysine** substitution at position 6 (E6K) and the presence of **hemoglobin C** (Hb C; called *sickle-hemoglobin C disease*), a Hb $S^{\beta+}$–thalassemia mutation, or a Hb $S^{\beta0}$–thalassemia mutation.

f.   **Clinical features include**: individuals healthy at birth; symptomatic later in infancy or childhood as fetal hemoglobin (Hb F) levels decrease; painful swelling of hands and feet (dactylitis); variable degrees of hemolysis; intermittent episodes of vascular occlusion resulting in ischemia and infarction of spleen, brain, lungs, and kidneys; frequent infections (e.g., pneumococcal sepsis or meningitis); and mean life expectancy is 30 years of age.

III   X-Linked Dominant Inheritance (Figure 5-1D; Table 5-1)

A.   INTRODUCTION. In X-linked dominant inheritance, the disease is observed **in both males and females (with no male-to-male transmission)**. All daughters of an affected man will be affected, because all receive the X chromosome bearing the mutant gene from the father. All sons of an affected man will be normal, because they receive only the Y chromosome from the father. Most X-linked dominant diseases are lethal in males.

B.   EXAMPLES OF X-LINKED DOMINANT DISEASES.

1.   Hypophosphatemic rickets (HR).

a.   HR is an X-linked dominant genetic disorder caused by various mutations in the *PHEX* **gene** on **chromosome Xp22.1** for <u>p</u>hosphate regulating <u>e</u>ndopeptidase on the <u>X</u> chromosome, which is a cell membrane–bound protein-cleaving enzyme that degrades **phosphatonins** (hormonelike circulating factors that increase PO_4^{3-} excretion and decrease bone mineralization).

b. HR is caused by missense, nonsense, small deletion, small insertion, or RNA splicing mutations. These mutations result in the inability of PHEX to degrade phosphatonins so that high circulating levels of phosphatonins occur, which causes increased PO_4^{3-} excretion and **decreased bone mineralization.** These mutations also result in the underexpression of $Na^+-PO_4^{3-}$ **cotransporter** in the kidney, which causes a **decreased PO_4^{3-} absorption.**

c. **Clinical features include**: a vitamin D–resistant rickets characterized by a low serum concentration of PO_4^{3-} and a high urinary concentration of PO_4^{3-} short stature, dental abscesses, early tooth decay, leg deformities that appeared at the time of weight bearing; and progressive departure from a normal growth rate.

2. Classic Rett syndrome (CRS).

a. CRS is an X-linked dominant genetic disorder caused by various mutations in the *MECP2* **gene** on **chromosome Xq28** for <u>methyl-C</u>pG-binding protein <u>2</u>, which has a methyl-binding domain (binds to 5-methylcytosine–rich DNA) and a transcription repression domain (recruits other proteins that repress transcription).

b. CRS is caused by missense, nonsense, and small deletion mutations. These mutations result in the inability of MECP to bind 5-methylcytosine–rich DNA and to repress transcription.

c. **Clinical features include**: a progressive neurologic disorder in girls where development from birth–18 months of age is normal; later, a short period of developmental stagnation is observed followed by rapid regression in language and motor skills; purposeful use of the hands is replaced by repetitive, stereotypic hand movements (hallmark); screaming fits; inconsolable crying; autism; and mental retardation.

IV. X-Linked Recessive Inheritance (Figure 5-1E; Table 5-1)

A. **INTRODUCTION.** In X-linked recessive inheritance, the disease is <u>usually</u> observed **only in the males (with no male-to-male transmission)**, since males have only one X chromosome; that is, males are **hemizygous** for X-linked genes (i.e., there is no backup copy of the gene). All daughters of affected males will be carriers (heterozygotes), and carrier females have a 50% risk of passing on the abnormal X with each pregnancy. In X-linked recessive inheritance, heterozygous females are clinically normal but may be detected by subtle clinical features (like intermediate enzyme levels, etc.). Can the disease ever be observed in females? The answer is yes because of the following two mechanisms:

1. In females, one of the two X chromosomes is inactivated during the **late blastocyst stage** to form a **Barr body** in a process called *dosage compensation (or lyonization)*. The choice of whether the maternally derived or paternally derived X chromosome becomes inactivated is a **random** and **permanent event**. The mechanism of dosage compensation involves **methylation of cytosine nucleotides.** If X chromosomes with the normal gene are inactivated in a sufficient number of cells, the female will have a large number of cells in which the one active X chromosome has the abnormal gene and may, therefore, be affected by the disease.

2. An X-linked recessive disease may also be observed in females who inherit both X chromosomes with the abnormal gene (i.e., **double dose**). In this case, the carrier mother and the affected father pass on the X chromosome with the abnormal gene. This used to be an extremely rare event, but with advances in treatment, more males affected with X-linked recessive diseases are surviving to reproductive age, so the probability of inheriting an abnormal X chromosome from an affected father is increasing.

B. EXAMPLE OF X-LINKED RECESSIVE DISEASE.

1. Duchenne muscular dystrophy (DMD).

    a. DMD is an X-linked recessive genetic disorder caused by various mutations in the *DMD* **gene** on **chromosome Xp21.2** for the **dystrophin**, which anchors the cytoskeleton (actin) of skeletal muscle cells to the extracellular matrix via a transmembrane protein (**α-dystrophin and β-dystrophin**), thereby stabilizing the cell membrane.

    b. DMD is caused by small deletion, large deletion, deletion of the entire gene, duplication of one of more exons, insertion, or single-based change mutations. These mutations result in absent/near absent dystrophin synthesis.

    c. **Clinical features include**: symptoms appear in early childhood with delays in sitting and standing independently; progressive muscle weakness and wasting; waddling gait; difficulty in climbing; wheelchair bound by 12 years of age; **Gowers maneuver** (patient rolls to the prone position, kneels, and pushes up to a standing position with hands against the knees and thighs); cardiomyopathy by 18 years of age; and death by ≈30 years of age due to cardiac or respiratory failure.

Ⅴ **The Family Pedigree in Various Inherited Diseases (Figure 5-1)** A family pedigree is a graphic method of charting the family history by using various symbols.

Ⅵ **Selected Photographs of Mendelian Inherited Disorders (Figure 5-2)**

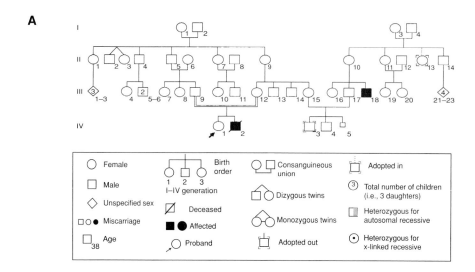

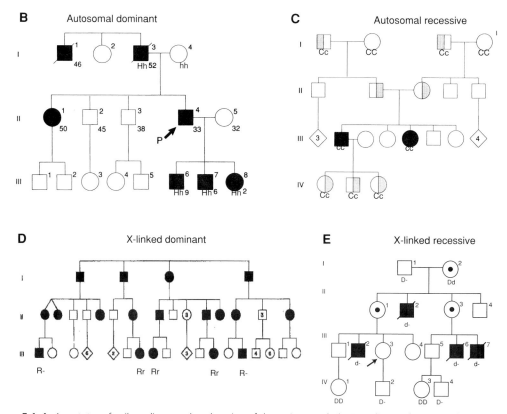

● **Figure 5-1 A:** A prototype family pedigree and explanation of the various symbols. **B:** Pedigree of autosomal dominant inheritance. The disease is observed **with equal probability in both males and females** who are **heterozygous for the mutant gene**. The characteristic pedigree is **vertical,** in that the disease is passed from one generation to the next. **C:** Pedigree of autosomal recessive inheritance. The disease is observed **with equal probability in both males and females** who are **homozygous for the mutant gene**. The characteristic pedigree is **horizontal,** in that affected individuals tend to be limited to a single sibship and the disease is not found in multiple generations. **D:** Pedigree of X-linked dominant inheritance. The disease is observed **in both males and females (with no male-to-male transmission).** All daughters of an affected man will be affected, because all receive the X chromosome bearing the mutant gene from the father. All sons of an affected man will be normal, because they receive only the Y chromosome from the father. **E:** Pedigree of X-linked recessive inheritance. The disease is <u>usually</u> observed **only in the males (with no male-to-male transmission).**

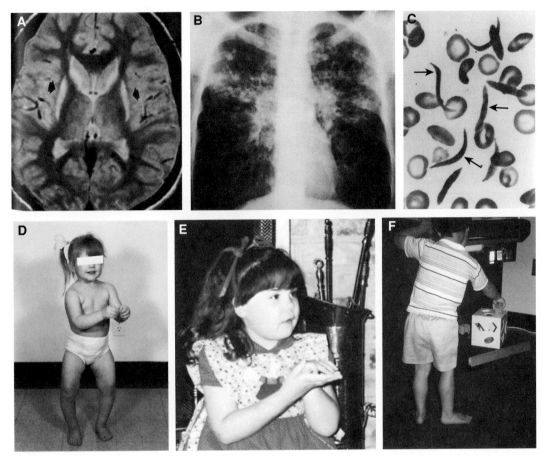

● **Figure 5-2 Selected photographs of mendelian inherited disorders. A:** Huntington disease. Magnetic resonance T2-weighted image shows high signal intensity in the globus pallidus (*arrows*). **B:** Cystic fibrosis. Posteroanterior
radiograph shows hyperinflation of both lungs, reduced size of the heart because of pulmonary compression, cyst formation, and atelectasis (collapse of alveoli) in both lungs. **C:** Sickle cell disease. Light micrograph shows sickle-shaped
red blood cells (drepanocytes; *arrows*). **D:** Hypophosphatemic rickets. A young girl with typical bowing of the legs. **E:**
Rett syndrome. A 5-year-old girl with the typical hand position that is characteristic of this disorder. **F:** Duchenne muscular dystrophy. A young boy with pseudohypertrophy of the calves. Note how the boy braces himself by grabbing onto
nearby furniture with his left hand. These patients are often late walkers.

TABLE 5-1	PARTIAL LIST OF SINGLE GENE INHERITED DISEASE BY TYPE	

Autosomal Dominant	Autosomal Recessive	X-Linked
Achondroplasia	α_1-Antitrypsin deficiency	**Dominant**
Acrocephalosyndactyly	Adrenogenital syndromes	Goltz syndrome
Adult polycystic kidney disease	Albinism	Hypophosphatemic rickets
Alport syndrome	Alpha thalassemia	Rett syndrome
Apert syndrome	Alkaptonuria	Incontinentia pigmenti
Bor syndrome	Argininosuccinic aciduria	Orofaciodigital
Brachydactyly	Ataxia telangiectasia	syndrome
Charcot-Marie-Tooth disease	Beta thalassemia	
Cleidocranial dysplasia	Bloom syndrome	**Recessive**
Crouzon craniofacial dysplasia	Branched chain ketonuria	Duchenne muscular
Craniostenosis	Childhood polycystic kidney disease	dystrophy
Diabetes associated	Cystic fibrosis	Ectodermal dysplasia
with defects in genes	Cystinuria	Ehlers-Danlos
for glucokinase,	Dwarfism	(type IX)
HNF-1α, and HNF-4α	Ehlers-Danlos syndrome (type VI)	Fabry disease
Ehlers-Danlos syndrome	Erythropoietic porphyria	Fragile X syndrome
(type IV)	Fanconi anemia	G6PD deficiency
Epidermolysis bullosa	Friedreich Ataxia	Hemophilia A & B
simplex	Fructosuria	Hunter syndrome
Familial adenomatous	Galactosemia	Ichthyosis
polyposis	Glycogen storage disease	Kennedy syndrome
Familial	Von Gierke (type Ia)	Kinky hair syndrome
hypercholesterolemia	Pompe (type II)	Lesch-Nyhan
(type IIa)	Cori (type IIIa)	syndrome
Goldenhar syndrome	Andersen (type IV)	Testicular
Heart-Hand syndrome	McArdle (type V)	feminization
Hereditary nonpolyposis	Hers (type VI)	Wiskott-Aldrich
colorectal cancer	Tarui (type VIII)	syndrome
Hereditary spherocytosis	Hemoglobin C disease	
Huntington disease	Hepatolenticular degeneration	
Marfan syndrome	Histidinemia	
Monilethrix	Homocystinuria	
Myotonic dystrophy 1 & 2	Hypophosphatasia	
Neurofibromatosis	Hypothyroidism	
Noonan syndrome	Junctional epidermolysis bullosa	
Osteogenesis imperfecta	Juvenile myoclonus epilepsy	
(types I & IV)	Lawrence Moon syndrome	
Pfeiffer syndrome	Lysosomal storage diseases	
Piebaldism	Tay Sachs	
Retinoblastoma	Gaucher	
Treacher Collins syndrome	Niemann-Pick	
Spinocerebellar ataxia	Krabbe	
1,2,3,6,7,8,11,17	Sandhoff	
Uncombable hair syndrome	Schindler	
Von Willebrand disease	GM1 gangliosidosis	
	Metachromatic leukodystrophy	

TABLE 5-1	PARTIAL LIST OF SINGLE GENE INHERITED DISEASE BY TYPE *(Continued)*	
Autosomal Dominant	**Autosomal Recessive**	**X-Linked**
Waardenburg syndrome	Mucopolysaccharidoses	
Williams-Beuren syndrome	Hurler	
	Sanfilippo A–D	
	Morquio A & B	
	Maroteaux-Lamy	
	Sly	
	Osteogenesis imperfecta (types II & III)	
	Oculocutaneous albinism (types I & II)	
	Peroxisomal disorders	
	Phenylketonuria	
	Premature senility	
	Pyruvate kinase deficiency	
	Retinitis pigmentosa	
	Sickle cell anemia	
	Trichothiodystrophy	
	Tyrosinemia	
	Xeroderma pigmentosa	

Chapter 6

Uniparental Disomy and Trinucleotide Repeats

Uniparental Disomy (UPD; Figure 6-1). UPD occurs when both copies of a chromosome are inherited from the same parent (sometimes UPD is only for a segment of a chromosome). If one copy is an identical copy of one homolog of a chromosome from a parent, then this is called *isodisomy*. If the parent passes on both homologs of a chromosome, then this is termed *heterodisomy*. In both cases, the child does not receive a copy of that chromosome from the other parent.

A. CAUSES.
   1. UPD can be caused by the loss of one chromosome from a cell where there is a trisomy for that particular chromosome ("**trisomy rescue**").
   2. UPD can also be caused when a gamete with two copies of a chromosome combines with a gamete with no copies of that chromosome.

B. DISEASES. UPD can be a factor in the causation of a number of diseases.
   1. **Prader-Willi and Angelman (PW/A) syndromes.**
      a. Since these diseases are mostly due to a microdeletion on chromosome 15, they are discussed in Chapter 11, but because this region involved is under control of genomic imprinting, UPD can cause these syndromes. Genomic imprinting is where the expression of a gene or genes depends on the parent of origin.
      b. If the PW/A region is deleted on paternal chromosome 15, then Prader-Willi syndrome results. UPD for maternal chromosome 15 is effectively a deletion of the paternal PW/A region, which results in Prader-Willi syndrome.
      c. If the PW/A region is deleted on maternal chromosome 15, then Angelman syndrome results. UPD for paternal chromosome 15 is effectively a deletion of the maternal PW/A region, which results in Angelman syndrome.
   2. **Beckwith-Wiedemann syndrome** can also be caused by UPD where there is an excess of paternal material or loss of maternal material at chromosome 11p15. This is also discussed in Chapter 11 IIB.
   3. **Autosomal recessive disorders.** In some cases, autosomal recessive disorders can be caused by UPD. Although this is a rare occurrence, UPD should be considered when only one parent is a carrier. For example, cystic fibrosis (CF) is an autosomal recessive disease, so both copies of the allele must have a mutation for the disease to be manifested. In UPD cases, the children have CF because they received the two mutations from the same parent.

Unstable Expanding Repeat Mutations (Dynamic Mutations)

   A. Dynamic mutations are mutations that involve the **expansion of a repeat sequence** either outside or inside the gene.

B. Dynamic mutations represent a new class of mutation in humans for which there is no counterpart in other organisms. The exact mechanism by which dynamic mutations occurs is not known.

C. Although dynamic mutations may occur during mitosis resulting in mosaicism, dynamic mutations often occur only during meiosis producing the female or male gametes.

D. THRESHOLD LENGTH. Dynamic mutations demonstrate a **threshold length. Below a certain threshold length**, the repeat sequence is stable, does not cause disease, and is propagated to successive generations without change in length. **Above a certain threshold length**, the repeat sequence is unstable, causes disease, and is propagated to successive generations in expanding lengths.

E. ANTICIPATION. Dynamic mutations demonstrate anticipation. Anticipation is one of the hallmarks of diseases caused by dynamic mutations. Anticipation means that a genetic disorder displays an **earlier age of onset** and/or a **greater degree of severity** in successive generations of the family pedigree.

F. PREMUTATION STATUS. A normal person may have certain number of repeats that have a high likelihood of being expanded during meiosis (i.e., a permutation status) such that his offspring are at increased risk of inheriting the disease.

G. Most of dynamic mutation diseases are caused by expansion of trinucleotide repeats, although longer repeats do play a role in some diseases. Dynamic mutations are divided into two categories: highly expanded repeats outside the gene and moderately expanded CAG repeats inside the gene.

Ⅲ Highly Expanded Repeats Outside the Gene.
In this category of dynamic mutation, various repeat sequences (e.g., CGG, CCG, GAA, CTG, CCTG, ATTCT, or CCCCGC-CCCGCG) undergo very large expansions. Below threshold length expansions are $\approx$5–50 repeats. Above threshold length expansions are $\approx$100–1,000 repeats. This category of dynamic mutations is characterized by the clinical conditions discussed next.

A. FRAGILE X SYNDROME (Martin-Bell Syndrome).
   1. **Fragile X syndrome** is an X-linked recessive genetic disorder caused by a 200–1,000+ unstable repeat sequence of $(CGG)_n$ outside the *FMR1* **gene on chromosome X** for the **fragile X mental retardation protein 1 (FMRP1)**, which is a nucleocytoplasmic shuttling protein that binds several messenger RNAs (mRNAs) found abundantly in neurons.
   2. The 200–1,000+ unstable repeat sequence of $(CGG)_n$ creates a fragile site on chromosome X, which is observed when cells are cultured in a **folate-depleted** medium. The 200–1,000+ unstable repeat sequence of $(CGG)_n$ has also been associated with **hypermethylation** of the *FMR1* gene so that FMRP1 is not expressed, which may lead to the phenotype of fragile X.
   3. Fragile X syndrome involves two mutation sites. **Fragile X site A** involves a 200–1,000+ unstable repeat sequence of $(CGG)_n$ located in a 5′ untranslated region (UTR) of the *FMR1* **gene** on **chromosome Xq27.3. Fragile X site B** involves a 200+ unstable repeat sequence of $(CCG)_n$ located in a promoter region of the *FMR1* **gene** on **chromosome Xq28.**

4. Normal *FMR1* alleles have ≈5–40 repeats. They are stably transmitted without any decrease or increase in repeat number.
5. Premutation *FMR1* alleles have ≈59–200 repeats. They are not stably transmitted. Females with permutation *FMR1* alleles are at risk for having children with fragile X syndrome.
6. **Prevalence.** The prevalence of fragile X syndrome is 1 in 4,000 males and 1 in 2,000 females.
7. **Clinical features include**: mental retardation (most severe in males); macroorchidism (postpubertal); speech delay; behavioral problems (e.g., hyperactivity, attention deficit); prominent forehead and jaw; joint laxity; and large, dysmorphic ears. Fragile X syndrome is the second leading cause of inherited mental retardation (Down syndrome is the number one cause).

B. FRIEDREICH ATAXIA (FRDA).

1. FRDA is an autosomal recessive genetic disorder caused by a 600–1,200 unstable repeat sequence of $(GAA)_n$ in intron 1 of the *FXN* gene on **chromosome 9q13-a21.1** for the **frataxin** protein, which is located on the inner mitochondrial membrane and plays a role in the synthesis of respiratory chain complexes I–III, mitochondrial iron content, and antioxidation defense.
2. A long-standing hypothesis is that FRDA is a result of mitochondrial accumulation of iron, which may promote oxidative stress injury.
3. Normal *FXN* alleles have ≈5–33 repeats. They are stably transmitted without any decrease or increase in repeat number.
4. Premutation *FXN* alleles have ≈34–65 repeats. They are not stably transmitted. Expansion of the permutation *FXN* alleles occurs in meiosis during the production of both sperm (paternal transmission) and ova (maternal transmission), since ≈96% of FRDA individuals are homozygous for the 600–1,200 unstable repeat sequence of $(GAA)_n$.
5. **Prevalence.** The prevalence of FRDA is 1 in 50,000.
6. **Clinical features include**: degeneration of the posterior columns and spinocerebellar tracts; loss of sensory neurons in the dorsal root ganglion; slowly progressive ataxia of all four limbs, with onset at 10–15 years of age; optic nerve atrophy; scoliosis; bladder dysfunction; swallowing dysfunction; pyramidal tract disease; cardiomyopathy (arrhythmias); and diabetes.

C. MYOTONIC DYSTROPHY TYPE 1 (DM1).

1. DM1 is an autosomal dominant genetic disorder caused by a >35–1,000 unstable repeat sequence of $(CTG)_n$ in the 3′ UTR of the *DMPK* gene on **chromosome 19q13.2-q13.3** for **myotonin-protein kinase,** which is a serine-threonine protein kinase associated with intercellular conduction and impulse transmission in the heart and skeletal muscle.
2. A hypothesis is that DM1 is caused by a gain-of-function RNA mechanism in which the alternate splicing of other genes (e.g., Cl^- ion channels, insulin receptor) occurs.
3. Normal *DMPK* alleles have ≈5–35 repeats. They are stably transmitted without any decrease or increase in repeat number.
4. Premutation *DMPK* alleles have ≈35–49 repeats. They are not stably transmitted. Individuals with permutation *DMPK* alleles are at risk for having children with DM1. A child with severe DM1 (i.e., congenital DM1) most frequently inherits the expanded repeat from the mother.

5. **Prevalence.** The prevalence of DM1 is 1 in 100,000 children in Japan; 1 in 10,000 in Iceland; and 1 in 20,000 worldwide.

6. **Clinical features include**: muscle weakness and wasting, myotonia (delayed muscle relaxation after contraction), cataracts, cardiomyopathy with conduction defects, multiple endocrinopathies, onset at 20–30 years of age, and low intelligence or dementia.

D. **SPINOCEREBELLAR ATAXIA (SCA 8 and SCA 11).** Numerous classification systems have been proposed for the autosomal dominant ataxias. Using a system based on genetic loci, numerous SCAs have been classified (SCA1–26; numbers continue to grow). SCA involves multiple mutation sites and a heterogeneous group of repeat sequences. Clinical features include increasing cerebellar ataxia.

IV Moderately Expanded CAG Repeats Inside the Gene. In this category of dynamic mutation, a CAG repeat sequences undergoes moderate expansions. Below-threshold length expansions are ≈10–30 repeats. Above-threshold length expansions are ≈40–200 repeats. Since CAG codes for the amino acid **glutamine**, a long tract of glutamines (**polyglutamine tract**) will be inserted into the amino acid sequence of the protein and causes the protein to aggregate within certain cells. This category of dynamic mutations is characterized by the clinical conditions discussed next.

A. **HUNTINGTON DISEASE (HD) (See Chapter 5 IG1).**

B. **SPINAL AND BULBAR MUSCULAR ATROPHY (SBMA; Kennedy Syndrome).**
1. SBMA is an X-linked recessive genetic disorder caused by a >38 repeat sequence of $(CAG)_n$ in the coding sequence of the *AR* **gene** on **chromosome Xq11-q12** for the **androgen receptor**, which is a member of the steroid-thyroid-retinoid superfamily of nuclear receptors and expressed in the brain, spinal cord, and muscle.
2. A hypothesis is that SBMA is caused by a gain-of-function mutation, because there is a well-known syndrome called *complete androgen insensitivity* that is caused by a loss-of-function mutation in the *AR* gene.
3. Normal *AR* alleles have ≤34 repeats.
4. Premutation *AR* alleles have not been reported to date.
5. **Prevalence.** The prevalence of SBMA is <1 in 50,000 live males in the white and Asian population. SBMA occurs only in males.
6. **Clinical features include**: progressive loss of anterior motor neurons, proximal muscle weakness, muscle atrophy, muscle fasciculations, difficulty in swallowing and speech articulation, late-onset gynecomastia, defective spermatogenesis with reduced fertility, testicular atrophy, and a hormonal profile consistent with androgen resistance.

C. **SPINOCEREBELLAR ATAXIA TYPE 3 (SCA3; Machado-Joseph Disease).**
1. SCA3 is an autosomal dominant genetic disorder caused by a 52–86 repeat sequence of $(CAG)_n$ in coding sequence of the *ATXN3* **gene** on **chromosome 14q24.3-q31** for the **ataxin 3** protein, which is a ubiquitin-specific protease that binds and cleaves ubiquitin chains and thereby participates in protein quality control pathways in the cell.
2. A hypothesis is that SCA3 is caused by impaired protein clearance, since mutant ataxin 3 forms nuclear inclusions that contain elements of the refolding and degradation machinery of the cell (i.e., chaperone and proteosome subunits).

3. Normal *ATXN3* alleles have ≤44 repeats.
4. Premutation *ATXN3* alleles have not been reported to date.
5. **Prevalence.** The prevalence of SCA3 in not known. Using a system based on genetic loci, numerous autosomal dominant ataxias have been classified (SCA1-26) and the numbers continue to grow. In general, all autosomal dominant ataxias are rare.
6. **Clinical features include**: progressive cerebellar ataxia, dysarthria, bulbar dysfunction, extrapyramidal features including rigidity and dystonia, upper and lower motor neuron signs, cognitive impairments, onset at 20–50 years of age, individuals becoming wheelchair-bound, and the finding of nuclear inclusions.

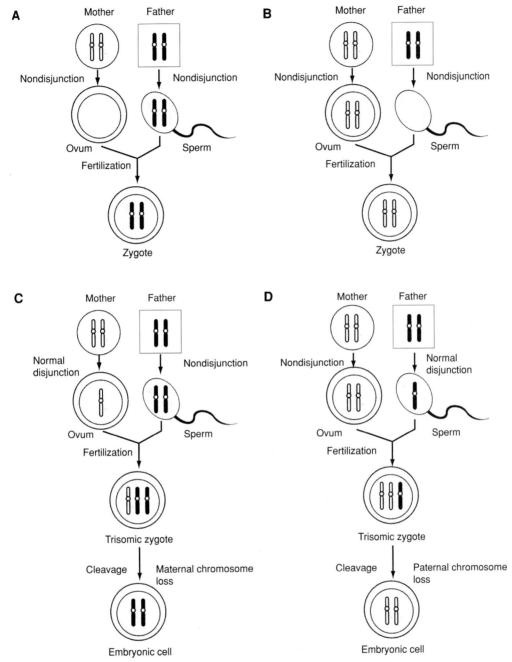

● **Figure 6-1 Uniparental disomy. A:** Maternal nondisjunction produces an ovum with no copies of a specific chromosome, and paternal nondisjunction produces a sperm with two copies of the same chromosome. After fertilization, the zygote has no copies of the maternal chromosome and two copies of the paternal chromosome. **B:** Maternal nondisjunction produces an ovum with two copies of a specific chromosome, and paternal nondisjunction produces a sperm with no copies of the same chromosome. After fertilization, the zygote has two copies of the maternal chromosome and no copies of the paternal chromosome. **C:** Maternal disjunction produces an ovum with one copy of a specific chromosome, and paternal nondisjunction produces a sperm with two copies of the same chromosome. After fertilization, the zygote has three copies of the same chromosome (i.e., a trisomic zygote). The maternal chromosome is lost during mitosis of the cleavage stage, which produces embryonic cells with two copies of the paternal chromosome. **D:** Maternal nondisjunction produces an ovum with two copies of a specific chromosome, and paternal disjunction produces a sperm with one copy of the same chromosome. After fertilization, the zygote has three copies of the same chromosome (i.e., a trisomic zygote). The paternal chromosome is lost during mitosis of the cleavage stage, which produces embryonic cells with two copies of the maternal chromosome. (Maternal chromosomes, white; paternal chromosomes, black.)

Chapter 7

Multifactorial Inherited Diseases

Ⅰ Introduction. Multifactorial inheritance involves many genes that have an additive effect (**genetic component**) interacting with the environment (**environmental component**). Both components contribute to a person inheriting the liability to develop a certain disease. If only the genetic component of a multifactorial disease is considered, the term *polygenic* ("many genes") is used. Inheritance patterns in multifactorial diseases usually do not conform to those seen with mendelian or cytogenetic inheritance. Recurrence risks are based on empiric data from population studies.

Ⅱ Classes of Multifactorial Traits

A. QUANTITATIVE TRAITS (Figure 7-1A). These traits are determined by many different genes along with environmental factors (e.g., diet) that determine the phenotypic outcome. These phenotypic traits tend to follow a normal distribution in the population. Some examples include: height, weight, blood pressure, and intelligence.

B. THRESHOLD TRAITS (Figure 7-1B).
  1. These traits are relatively common, isolated congenital defects with an underlying variation in **liability**. Liability is the predisposition for a malformation that may be determined by more than one gene. Liability can vary based on gender.
  2. In threshold traits, there is a liability distribution where a clinical effect is not seen until the threshold is reached. Individuals above this threshold have the defect because they have more of the alleles and environmental factors that cause the defect than those below the threshold.
  3. Some examples of congenital defects that follow this model are: isolated cleft lip and/or cleft palate, neural tube defects (spina bifida and anencephaly), club foot, and pyloric stenosis. An example of an environmental component to a threshold trait is neural tube defects, where increased folic acid intake before and during pregnancy helps to prevent spina bifida and anencephaly.

C. COMMON DISEASES. These are generally disorders of adult life in which environmental factors play a role, but there definitely is a genetic contribution. Some examples include: cancer, diabetes mellitus, hypertension, heart disease, alcoholism, and psychiatric disorders (e.g., Alzheimer disease, schizophrenia, bipolar disorder).

Ⅲ Factors Affecting Recurrence Risks. The risk for having a multifactorial genetic disease is the empirically derived population risk. However, if an individual in a family has a multifactorial condition, there are a number of factors that influence the risk of its recurrence in that family.

A. **HERITABILITY.** Heritability (H) is the estimate of the contribution that genetic factors make to a trait. If H = 0, then the observed phenotypic variation is entirely due to environmental factors. If H = 1, then the observed phenotypic variation is entirely due to genetic factors (0, environmental factors → 1, genetic factors). For example, a heritability of 0.80 indicates a strong genetic input to the expression of a phenotype in the particular population under study. The higher the concordance (both having the same trait) of a trait in monozygotic (MZ) twins versus dizygotic (DZ) twins, the higher the heritability (↑concordance = ↑heritability). This is indicated in the following examples.

  1. The concordance for idiopathic seizure is 85%–90% in MZ twins versus 10%–15% in DZ twins. This means that idiopathic seizure has a high heritability (**85%–90% in MZ twins vs. 10%–15% in DZ twins = ↑H**).

  2. The concordance for cleft palate is 25% in MZ twins versus 10% in DZ twins. This means that cleft palate has a low heritability (**25% in MZ vs. 10% in DZ = ↓H**).

B. **INCIDENCE IN THE POPULATION.** The incidence of a trait often varies between populations. In Ireland, the incidence of neural tube defects is 1 in 200 births. In the United States, the incidence of neural tube defects is 1 in 1,000 births. The recurrence risk in first-degree relatives is approximately the square root of the population incidence (**risk of recurrence = √ population incidence**).

C. **SEX BIAS.**

  1. Multifactorial diseases/malformations are often more common in one sex than in the other (i.e., sex-biased). In sex-biased diseases/malformations, the recurrence risk is higher in the following two conditions:

    a. If an affected child in the family is of the more-affected sex, then the recurrence risk to a same-sexed sibling is higher than the recurrence risk to another-sex sibling. The risk to either-sex sibling is greater than the general population risk for the condition.

    b. If an affected child in the family is of the less-affected sex, then the recurrence risk to another-sexed sibling is higher than the recurrence risk to a same-sexed sibling. The risk to either-sex sibling is greater than the general population risk for the condition.

  2. Examples of male sex-biased diseases/malformations include: pyloric stenosis, cleft lip with or without cleft palate, spina bifida, and anencephaly. Examples of female sex-biased diseases/malformations include: congenital hip dysplasia and idiopathic scoliosis.

    a. *Example*: **Male-biased pyloric stenosis.** Pyloric stenosis is an obstruction of the area between the stomach and the intestines that causes severe feeding problems and is more common in males (male-biased).

      i. If a male child in a family is born with pyloric stenosis, then the recurrence risk to his future brother is 3.8%, whereas the recurrence risk to his future sister is 2.7%.
      However,

      ii. If a female child in a family is born with pyloric stenosis, then the recurrence risk to her future brother is 9.2%, whereas the recurrence risk to her future sister is 3.8%.

    b. *Example*: **Female-biased idiopathic scoliosis.** Idiopathic scoliosis is a lateral deviation of the vertebral column that involves both deviations and rotation of the vertebral bodies due to unknown causes.

    i. If a female child in a family is born with idiopathic scoliosis, then the recurrence risk to her future sister is 5.3%, whereas the recurrence risk to her future brother is 1.1%.
However,

    ii. If a male child in a family is born with idiopathic scoliosis, then the recurrence risk to his future sister is 7.5%, whereas the recurrence risk to his future brother is 5.4%.

D. DEGREE OF RELATIONSHIP. The recurrence risk decreases as the remoteness of relationship to the proband increases (↓**recurrence risk as** ↑**remoteness**). For example, in cleft palate, the recurrence risk is:
1. 4.0% for first-degree relatives.
2. 0.7% for second-degree relatives.
3. 0.3% for third-degree relatives, which is close to the population incidence.

E. NUMBER OF AFFECTED RELATIVES. The recurrence risk increases as the number of affected relatives increases (↑**recurrence risk as** ↑**number of affected relatives**). This is because multiple affected relatives suggest a high liability in the family for a multifactorial trait. For example, in cleft lip and cleft palate, the recurrence risk is:
1. 4% after having one affected child.
2. 10% after having two affected children.

F. SEVERITY OF THE DISORDER. The recurrence risk increases as the severity of the disorder increases (↑**recurrence risk as** ↑**severity of disorder**). This is because a more severely affected individual suggests a high liability for the trait. For example, in bilateral cleft lip and cleft palate, the recurrence risk is:
1. 2.5% after having a child with unilateral cleft lip.
2. 5.6% after having a child with bilateral cleft lip and cleft palate.

G. CONSANGUINITY (Kinship).
1. The risk of having a child with a birth defect increases as the consanguinity of the mating partners increases (↑**risk as** ↑**consanguinity**). This is because close consanguinity mating partners have high likelihood of sharing predisposing genes (i.e., a genetic relationship).
2. For example, if the mating partners are first cousins, the risk of having a child with a birth defect is 6%–10% whereas the general population risk of having a child with a birth defect is 3%–5%.

IV Some Common Multifactorial Conditions

A. TYPE 1 DIABETES.
1. The characteristic dysfunction in this disease is a **destruction of pancreatic beta cells** that produce insulin, which results clinically in hyperglycemia, ketoacidosis, and exogenous insulin dependence.
2. Long-term clinical effects include neuropathy, retinopathy leading to blindness, and nephropathy leading to kidney failure.
3. Type 1 diabetes demonstrates an association with the highly polymorphic *HLA class II* (human leukocyte antigen) genes, which play a role in immune responsiveness. The specific loci involved in type 1 diabetes are called *HLA-DR3* and *HLA-DR4 loci*. HLA-DR3 and HLA-DR4 loci are located on the **short arm (p arm) of chromosome 6 (p6)**. HLA-DR3 and HLA-DR4 loci code for **cell-surface glycoproteins** that are

structurally similar to immunoglobulin proteins and are expressed mainly by B lymphocytes and macrophages.

4. It is **hypothesized** that alleles closely linked to HLA-DR3 and HLA-DR4 loci somehow alter the immune response such that the individual has an immune response to an environmental antigen (e.g., virus). The immune response "spills over" and leads to the destruction of pancreatic beta cells. Markers for immune destruction of pancreatic beta cells include **autoantibodies to glutamic acid decarboxylase (GAD_{65}), insulin,** and **tyrosine phosphatases IA-2 and IA-2β.**

5. The heritability of type 1 diabetes is 0.35–0.50, which indicates that there is a relatively weak genetic component to type 1 diabetes and that environmental factors (e.g., viruses or other environmental antigens) play a role. The MZ twin concordance rate is 35%–50%. The sibling recurrence risk is 1%–6%.

B. TYPE 2 DIABETES.

1. Type 2 diabetes accounts for ≈90% of all cases of diabetes. In contrast to type 1 diabetes, there is almost always some insulin production. Type 2 diabetics develop insulin resistance, a condition where the cells have reduced ability to use insulin.

2. The disease typically occurs in adults over 40 years of age, with the greatest risk factors being obesity, diet, and family history.

3. The heritability of type 2 diabetes is 0.90, which indicates that there is a strong genetic component to type 2 diabetes and that environmental factors (e.g., obesity, diet) play a role. The MZ twin concordance rate is 90%. The sibling recurrence risk 10%–40%. Populations that have adopted Western diet and activity patterns show an increased incidence of the disease, most likely due to an increase in obesity.

4. A number of genes have been linked to type 2 diabetes, but the genetic component of the disease is not completely understood.

C. HYPERTENSION.
Hypertension is a major factor in cardiovascular disease and strokes. Although a number of genes have been linked to hypertension, hypertension involves complex physiologic processes that involve many genes. The role of environmental factors is also recognized in the etiology of hypertension (e.g., sodium in the diet, physical activity, and weight gain). The heritability of hypertension is 0.20–0.40, which indicates that there is a relatively weak genetic component to hypertension and that environmental factors play a role.

D. HEART DISEASE.
Some genes that are known to play a role in heart disease are involved with the regulation of lipoproteins in the circulation. There are a number of risk factors for heart disease (e.g., cigarette smoking, obesity, hypertension, high cholesterol, and a positive family history). The risk of developing heart disease increases in an individual who has the following:

1. A first-degree affected male relative (risk = ≈2 times the general population risk).
2. A first-degree affected female (least affected sex) relative (risk = >2 times the general population risk).
3. Many affected relatives (risk = >2 times the general population risk).
4. Affected relative or relatives who were diagnosed with heart disease at <55 years of age (risk = >2 times the general population risk).

E. CANCER.

1. Cancers can generally be considered as genetic diseases, but most of them are not strictly inherited. The fact that cancers tend to cluster in families demonstrates that there is a genetic component to the diseases as a group. The family clustering is

probably due to both shared genes that create a predisposition and shared environmental factors that trigger the cancer-causing event (e.g., a mutation of a proto-oncogene into an oncogene or a loss-of-function mutation of a tumor suppressor gene).

2. For example, the risk of developing breast cancer doubles for first-degree relatives of women diagnosed with the disease. The risk also increases if more than one first-degree relative has breast cancer and increases even more if the cancers developed relatively early (before the age of 45). However, the genetic components of many cancers are poorly understood.

3. The role of some proto-oncogenes and tumor suppressor genes in the etiology of cancer is indicated in Table 7-1 and 7-2.

4. The role of environmental and infectious factors in the etiology of cancer is indicated in Table 7-3.

F.   CANCER EXAMPLES (Figure 7-1).

1.   Hereditary retinoblastoma (RB).

a.   Hereditary RB is an autosomal dominant genetic disorder caused by a mutation in the *RB1* gene on **chromosome 13q14.1** for the **RB protein**. More than 1,000 different mutations of the *RB1* gene have been identified, which include missense, frameshift, and RNA splicing mutations that result in a premature STOP codon and a **loss-of-function mutation**.

b.   RB protein binds to E2F (a gene regulatory protein) such that there will be no expression of target genes whose gene products stimulate the cell cycle at the G1 checkpoint. RB protein belongs to the family of **tumor suppressor genes**.

c.   Hereditary RB-affected individuals inherit one mutant copy of the *RB1* gene from their parents (an inherited germline mutation) followed by a somatic mutation of the second copy of the *RB1* gene later in life.

d.   If a parent of the proband has RB due to a RB1 germline mutation, the risk to each sibling of the proband of inheriting the RB1 germline mutation is 50%.

e.   If a person has hereditary RB (bilateral tumors), the risk of passing the mutated gene to his or her children is 50%.

f.   **Clinical features include**: a malignant tumor of the retina develops in children <5 years of age, a whitish mass in the pupillary area behind the lens (leukokoria; the cat's eye), and strabismus.

2.   Neurofibromatosis type 1 (NF1; von Recklinghausen disease).

a.   NF1 is a relatively common autosomal dominant genetic disorder caused by a mutation in the *NF1* gene on **chromosome 17q11.2** for the **neurofibromin** protein. More than 500 different mutations of the *NF1* gene have been identified, including **missense, nonsense, frameshift, whole gene deletions, intragenic deletions**, and **RNA splicing mutations**, all of which result in a **loss-of-function mutation**.

b.   Neurofibromin down regulates **p21 ras oncoprotein**; therefore, the *NF1* gene belongs to the family of **tumor suppressor genes** and regulates cAMP levels.

c.   Of those individuals affected with NF1, ≈50% inherit a mutant gene from an affected parent, whereas ≈50% have a *de novo* mutation.

d.   If a parent of the proband has NF1, the risk to the siblings of the proband is 50%. If the parents of the proband are normal, the risk to the siblings of the proband is very low but greater than that of the general population since the possibility of germline mosaicism exists. If a person has a dominantly inherited form of NF1, the risk of passing the mutated gene to his or her children is 50%.

e.   **Clinical features include**: multiple neural tumors (called *neurofibromas*) that are widely dispersed over the body and reveal proliferation of all elements of a peripheral nerve including neurites, fibroblasts, and Schwann cells of neural crest origin; numerous pigmented skin lesions (called *café au lait spots*) probably associated with melanocytes of neural crest origin; axillary and inguinal freckling; scoliosis; vertebral dysplasia; and pigmented iris hamartomas (called *Lisch nodules*).

3. **BRCA1 and BRCA2 hereditary breast cancer**

   a. A predisposition to breast, ovarian, and prostate cancer may be associated with mutations in the *BRCA1* gene and *BRCA2* gene, although the exact percentage of risk is not known and even appears to be variable within families.

   b. BRCA1 and BRCA2 hereditary breast cancer is an autosomal genetic disorder caused by a mutation in the *BRCA1* gene on **chromosome 17q21** for the **breast cancer type 1 susceptibility protein** or a mutation in the *BRCA2* gene on **chromosome 13q12.3** for the **breast cancer type 2 susceptibility protein.**

   c. BRCA type 1 and type 2 susceptibility proteins bind RAD51 protein, which plays a role in **double-strand DNA break repair.**

   d. More than 600 different mutations of the *BRCA1* gene have been identified, all of which result in a **loss-of-function mutation.**

   e. More than 450 different mutations of the *BRCA2* gene have been identified, all of which result in a **loss-of-function mutation.**

   f. If a person has hereditary breast cancer, the risk of passing the mutated gene to his or her children is 50%.

   g. **Clinical features include:** early onset of breast cancer, bilateral breast cancer, family history of breast or ovarian cancer consistent with autosomal dominant inheritance, and a family history of male breast cancer.

4. **Familial adenomatous polyposis (FAP).**

   a. FAP is an autosomal dominant genetic disorder caused by a mutation in the **APC gene** on **chromosome 5q21-q22** for the **adenomatous polyposis coli protein.** More than 800 different germline mutations of the *APC* gene have been identified, all of which result in a **loss-of-function mutation.** The most common germline APC mutation is a **5-base pair deletion** at codon 1309.

   b. APC protein binds **glycogen synthase kinase 3b (GSK-3b),** which targets ß-catenin. APC protein maintains normal apoptosis and inhibits cell proliferation through the **Wnt signal transduction pathway,** therefore, APC belongs to the family of **tumor suppressor genes.**

   c. Of those individuals affected with FAP, ≈80% inherit a mutant gene from an affected parent, whereas ≈20% have a *de novo* mutation.

   d. If a parent of the proband has FAP due to an APC germline mutation, the risk to each sibling of the proband of inheriting the APC germline mutation is 50%.

   e. If a person has FAP due to an APC germline mutation, the risk of passing the mutated *APC* gene to his or her children is 50%.

   f. A majority of colorectal cancers develop slowly through a series of histopathologic changes, each of which has been associated with mutations of specific proto-oncogenes and tumor suppressor genes as follows: normal epithelium → a small polyp involves mutation of the *APC* tumor suppressor gene; small polyp → large polyp involves mutation of *ras* proto-oncogene; large polyp → carcinoma → metastasis involves mutation of the *DCC* tumor suppressor gene and the *p53* tumor suppressor gene.

   g. **Clinical features include:** colorectal adenomatous polyps appear at 7–35 years of age, inevitably leading to colon cancer; thousands of polyps can be observed in the colon; and gastric polyps may be present.

TABLE 7-1		PROTO-ONCOGENES[a] AND ASSOCIATED CANCERS	
Class	Protein Encoded by Proto-oncogene	Oncogene	Cancer
Growth factors	PDGF	*sis*	Astrocytoma, osteosarcoma
Receptors	EGFR	*erbB2*	Breast carcinoma (marker of aggressiveness)
Signal transducers	Tyrosine kinase	*abl/bcr*	CML t(9;22)(q34;q11); Philadelphia chromosome
	G-protein	*ras*[b]	Human bladder, lung, colon, and pancreas carcinomas
Transcription factors	Leucine zipper ProteinI	*fos*	Finkel-Biskes-Jinkins osteosarcoma
	Helix-loop-helix protein	N-*myc*	Neuroblastoma
	Helix-loop-helix protein	*myc*	Burkitt lymphoma t(8;14)(q24;q32)
	Retinoic acid receptor (zinc finger protein)	*pml/rarα*	APL t(15;17)(q22;q21)

PDGF, platelet-derived growth factor; EGFR, epidermal growth factor receptor; CML, chronic myeloid leukemia; APL, acute promyelocytic leukemia.

[a]Since the cell cycle can be regulated at many different points, it would be expected that proto-oncogenes would fall into many different classes. Consequently, proto-oncogenes have been classified in four classes (i.e., growth factors, receptors, signal transducers, and transcription factors) as indicated.

[b]The *ras* oncogene is found in about 15% of all human cancers, including 25% of lung cancers, 50% of colon cancers, and 90% of pancreatic cancers.

TABLE 7-2		TUMOR SUPPRESSOR GENES AND ASSOCIATED CANCERS
Tumor Suppressor Gene	Chromosome	Mutation of Tumor Suppressor Gene Involved in the Following Types of Cancer
RB1	13q14.1	Retinoblastoma; carcinomas of the breast, prostate, bladder, and lung
p53	17p13	Most human cancers, Li-Fraumeni syndrome
BRCA1[a]	17q21	Breast and ovarian cancer
BRCA2	13q12.3	Breast cancer
NF-1	17q12	Schwannoma, neurofibromatosis type 1
WT-2	11p15	Wilms tumor
VHL	3p25	Von Hippel–Lindau disease, retinal and cerebellar hemangioblastomas
APC	5q21-q22	Familial adenomatous polyposis coli, carcinomas of the colon
DCC	18	Carcinomas of the colon and stomach

RB, retinoblastoma; BRCA, breast cancer; NF-1, neurofibromatosis; WT, Wilms tumor; VHL, von Hippel–Lindau disease; APC, familial adenomatous polyposis coli; DCC, deleted in colon carcinoma.

[a]The BRCA1 tumor suppressor gene is located on chromosome 17q21 and encodes for normal BRCA protein (a zinc finger gene regulatory protein) containing phosphotyrosine that will suppress the cell cycle. A mutation of the *BRCA1* gene is present in 5%–10% of women with breast cancer and confers a very high lifetime risk of breast and ovarian cancer.

TABLE 7-3	ENVIRONMENTAL AND INFECTIOUS FACTORS IN CANCER
Factor	**Cancer**
Cigarette smoking (3-methylcholanthrene)	Squamous cell carcinoma of the lung
Asbestos	Pleural mesothelioma
Nitrosamines	Stomach carcinoma
Ultraviolet radiation	Melanoma, basal cell carcinoma, squamous carcinoma of the skin
Nulliparity	Breast cancer
Oral contraceptives	
Estrogen replacement therapy	
Low-fiber diet	Colorectal cancer
Nickel, silica, beryllium, chromium	Bronchogenic carcinoma
Benzene	Acute leukemia
Cyclophosphamide, ß-naphthylamine	Transitional cell carcinoma of the urinary bladder
Diethylstilbestrol	Clear cell carcinoma of the vagina
HPV	Carcinoma of the cervix
HHV 8	Kaposi sarcoma
HBV, HCV	Primary hepatocellular carcinoma
HTLV-1	T-cell leukemia and lymphoma

HPV, human papilloma virus; HHV 8, human herpesvirus 8; HBV, hepatitis B; HCV, hepatitis C; HTLV-1, human T-cell leukemia virus.

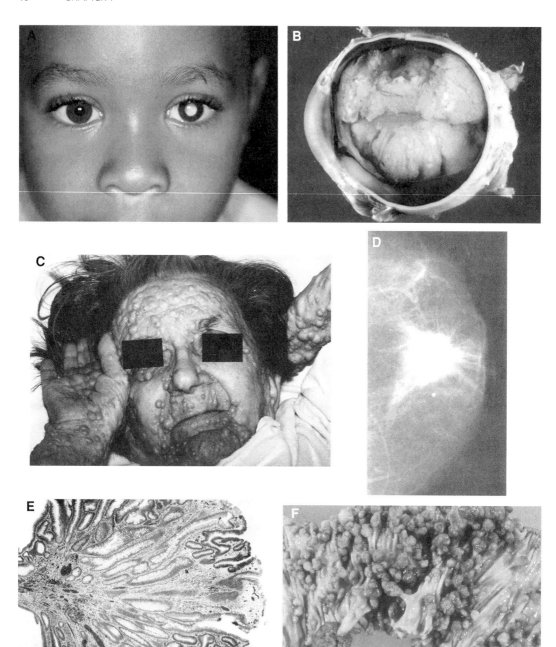

● **Figure 7-1 Cancer. Retinoblastoma (A, B).** Photograph shows a young child with a white pupil (leukokoria; cat's eye) in the left eye. **B:** Surgical specimen shows that the eye is almost completely filled with a cream-colored intraocular retinoblastoma. **C: Neurofibromatosis type I.** Photograph shows a woman with generalized neurofibromas on the face and arms. **D: Breast cancer.** Mammogram shows a malignant mass that has the following characteristics: shape is irregular with many lobulations; margins are irregular or spiculated; density is medium high; breast architecture may be distorted; and calcifications (not shown) are small, irregular, variable, and found within ducts (called *ductal casts*). **Familial adenomatous polyposis (E, F). E:** Light micrograph of an adenomatous polyp. A polyp is a tumorous mass that extends into the lumen of the colon. Note the convoluted, irregular arrangement of the intestinal glands with the basement membrane intact. **F:** Photograph shows a colon that contains thousands of adenomatous polyps.

Chapter 8

Mitochondrial Inheritance

I **Mitochondrial Function.** Mitochondria are involved in the production of acetyl coenzyme A (CoA), the tricarboxylic acid cycle, fatty acid b-oxidation, amino acid oxidation, oxidative phosphorylation (which causes the **synthesis of adenosine triphosphate [ATP]** driven by electron transfer to oxygen), and apoptosis. ATP is the energy source for cellular metabolism, which means that mitochondria are essential for cell functioning. There are ≈100 mitochondria/cell. However, different cell types have differing energy needs, so they require differing numbers of mitochondria.

A. Substrates are metabolized in the mitochondrial matrix to produce **acetyl CoA**, which is oxidized by the tricarboxylic acid cycle to carbon dioxide.

B. The energy released by this oxidation is captured by reduced nicotinamide adenine dinucleotide (NADH) and flavin adenine dinucleotide (FADH$_2$). NADH and FADH$_2$ are further oxidized, producing **hydrogen ions** and **electrons.**

C. The electrons are transferred along the **electron transport chain,** which is accompanied by the outward pumping of hydrogen ions into the intermembrane space (**chemiosmotic theory**). The electron transport chain includes the following enzymes: NADH dehydrogenase (complex I), succinate dehydrogenase (complex II), ubiquinone-cytochrome c oxidoreductase (complex III), and cytochrome oxidase (complex IV).

D. The **F$_0$ subunit of ATP synthase** forms a transmembrane hydrogen ion pore so that hydrogen ions can flow from the intermembrane space into the matrix, where the **F$_1$ subunit of ATP synthase** catalyzes the reaction **ADP + P$_i$ → ATP.**

II The Human Mitochondrial Genome (Figure 8-1)

A. The mitochondrial genome is completely separate from the nuclear genome. In this regard, transcription of mitochondrial DNA (mtDNA) occurs in the mitochondrial matrix, whereas transcription of nuclear DNA occurs in the nucleus.

B. The replication of mtDNA is catalyzed by **DNA polymerase γ**, whereas the replication of nuclear DNA is catalyzed by **DNA polymerase α and λ.**

C. There are several copies of the genome per mitochondrion.

D. The human mitochondrial genome consists of mtDNA arranged as a **circular piece of double-stranded DNA** (**H strand** and **L strand**) with 16,569 base pairs and is located within the **mitochondrial matrix.**

E.   In contrast to the human nuclear genome, mtDNA is not protected by histones (i.e., **histone-free**).

F.   The human mitochondrial genome codes for **37 genes** that make up ≈93% **of the human mitochondrial genome**. There are **13 protein-coding genes** and **24 RNA-coding genes**. The fact that the 37 genes make up ≈93% of the human mitochondrial genome means that ≈93% **of the human mitochondrial genome consists of coding DNA** and ≈7% **of the human mitochondrial genome consists of noncoding DNA** (compare with the human nuclear genome; Chapter 1).

G.   All human *mtDNA* **genes contain only exons** (i.e., no introns are present).

III The Protein-Coding Genes

A.   The protein-coding genes of the mitochondrial genome encode for **13 proteins** that are not complete enzymes but are **subunits of multimeric enzyme complexes** used in electron transport and ATP synthesis. These 13 proteins are synthesized on mitochondrial ribosomes.

B.   The 13 proteins include the following:
   1.   Seven subunits of the NADH dehydrogenase (i.e., ND1, ND2, ND3, ND4L, ND4, ND5, and ND6; complex I)
   2.   Three subunits of the cytochrome oxidase (i.e., CO1, CO2, and CO3; complex IV)
   3.   Two subunits of the F_0 ATPase (i.e., ATPsyn 6 and ATPsyn 8)
   4.   One subunit (cytochrome b) of ubiquinone-cytochrome c oxidoreductase (i.e., CYB1; complex III).

IV The RNA-Coding Genes

A.   The RNA-coding genes of the mitochondrial genome encode for **24 RNAs**.
B.   The 24 RNAs include the following:
   1.   Two rRNAs (16S and 23S)
   2.   Twenty-two tRNAs (corresponding to each amino acid)

V Other Mitochondrial Proteins.
All other mitochondrial proteins (e.g., enzymes of the citric acid cycle, DNA polymerase, RNA polymerase) are **encoded by about 90 genes in the nuclear DNA**, synthesized on cytoplasmic ribosomes, and then **imported into the mitochondria**.

VI Mutation Rate.
The mutation rate of mtDNA is about ten times that of nuclear DNA because only limited DNA repair mechanism exists in the mitochondrial matrix. This higher mutation rate may also be related to free radical production during oxidative phosphorylation.

VII Mitochondrial Inheritance (See Figure 8-1)

A.   In mitochondrial inheritance, the disease is observed in **both males and females who have an affected mother** (not father).

B. Diseases that have mitochondrial inheritance are caused by mutations in mtDNA. They are inherited entirely through **maternal transmission (maternally inherited)** because sperm mitochondria do not pass into the secondary oocyte at fertilization. Consequently, the mitochondrial genome of the zygote is determined exclusively by the mitochondria found in the cytoplasm of the unfertilized secondary oocyte.

C. Because mtDNA replicates autonomously from nuclear DNA and mitochondria segregate in daughter cells independently of nuclear chromosomes, the proportion of mitochondria carrying a mtDNA mutation can differ among somatic cells. This heterogeneity is termed *heteroplasmy* and plays a role in the variable phenotype of mitochondrial disease.

D. Mitochondria are the only cytoplasmic organelles in eukaryotic cells that show an inheritance independent of the nucleus (extranuclear inheritance).

E. The genes located on the circular mitochondrial chromosome have an exclusively maternal transmission pattern, whereas gene located on nuclear chromosomes have a mendelian inheritance patterns.

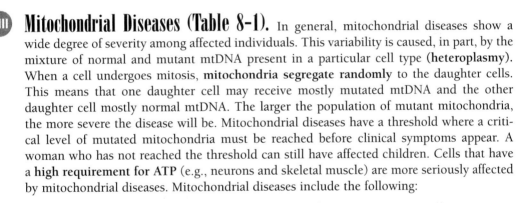 **Mitochondrial Diseases (Table 8-1).** In general, mitochondrial diseases show a wide degree of severity among affected individuals. This variability is caused, in part, by the mixture of normal and mutant mtDNA present in a particular cell type (**heteroplasmy**). When a cell undergoes mitosis, **mitochondria segregate randomly** to the daughter cells. This means that one daughter cell may receive mostly mutated mtDNA and the other daughter cell mostly normal mtDNA. The larger the population of mutant mitochondria, the more severe the disease will be. Mitochondrial diseases have a threshold where a critical level of mutated mitochondria must be reached before clinical symptoms appear. A woman who has not reached the threshold can still have affected children. Cells that have a **high requirement for ATP** (e.g., neurons and skeletal muscle) are more seriously affected by mitochondrial diseases. Mitochondrial diseases include the following:

A. LEBER HEREDITARY OPTIC NEUROPATHY (LHON).

  1. LHON is a mitochondrial genetic disorder caused by three mtDNA missense mutations, which account for 90% of all cases worldwide and are therefore designated as **primary LHON mutations.**

  2. The primary LHON mutations include:

   a. A mutation in the *ND4* gene (which encodes for subunit 4 of NADH dehydrogenase; complex I) whereby an A→G transition occurs at **nucleotide position 11778 (A11778G)**. This is the most common cause of LHON (≈50% of all cases).

   b. A mutation in the *ND1* gene (which encodes for subunit 1 of NADH dehydrogenase; complex I) whereby a G→A transition occurs at **nucleotide position 3460 (G3460A)**.

   c. A mutation in the *ND6* gene (which encodes for subunit 6 of NADH dehydrogenase; complex I) whereby a T→C transition occurs at **nucleotide position 14484 (T14484C)**.

  3. All three primary LHON mutations **decrease production of ATP** such that the demands of a very active neuronal metabolism cannot be met and suggest a common disease-causing mechanism.

  4. Heteroplasmy is rare, and expression of the disease is fairly uniform. Consequently, the family pedigree of LHON demonstrates a typical mitochondrial inheritance pattern.

5. **Clinical features include**: progressive optic nerve degeneration that results clinically in blindness, blurred vision, or loss of central vision; telangiectatic microangiopathy; disk pseudoedema; vascular tortuosity; onset occurs at ≈20 years of age with precipitous vision loss; and affect males far more often than females for some unknown reason.

B. MYOCLONIC EPILEPSY WITH RAGGED RED FIBERS SYNDROME (MERRF).

1. MERRF is a mitochondrial genetic disorder caused by a mutation in the $tRNA^{Lys}$ **gene** whereby an A→G transition occurs at **nucleotide position 8344 (A8344G)**.
2. The mutated $tRNA^{Lys}$ gene causes a **premature termination of translation** of the amino acid chain (the amount and the aminoacylation activity of the mutated $tRNA^{Lys}$ is not affected).
3. Mitochondrial enzymes with a large number of lysine residues will have a low probability of being completely synthesized. In this regard, **NADH dehydrogenase (complex I)** and **cytochrome oxidase (complex IV)**, both of which have a large number of lysine residues, have been shown to be synthesized at very low rates.
4. Heteroplasmy is common, and expression of the disease is highly variable.
5. Clinical features include myoclonus (muscle twitching), seizures, cerebellar ataxia, dementia, and mitochondrial myopathy (abnormal mitochondria within skeletal muscle that impart an irregular shape and blotchy red appearance to the muscle cells, hence the term *ragged red fibers*).

C. MITOCHONDRIAL MYOPATHY, ENCEPHALOPATHY, LACTIC ACIDOSIS, AND STROKELIKE EPISODES SYNDROME (MELAS).

1. MELAS is a mitochondrial genetic disorder caused by a mutation in the $tRNA^{Leu}$ **gene** whereby an A→G transition occurs at **nucleotide position 3243 (A3243G)**.
2. The mutated $tRNA^{Leu}$ gene causes a reduction in the amount and the aminoacylation of the mutated $tRNA^{Leu}$, a reduction in the association of mRNA with ribosomes, and altered incorporation of leucine into mitochondrial enzymes.
3. Mitochondrial enzymes with a large number of leucine residues will have a low probability of being completely synthesized. In this regard, cytochrome oxidase (complex IV) has been shown to be synthesized at very low rates.
4. Heteroplasmy is common, and expression of the disease is highly variable.
5. **Clinical features include**: mitochondrial myopathy, encephalopathy, lactic acidosis, and strokelike episodes.

D. KEARNS-SAYRE SYNDROME (KS).

1. KS is a mitochondrial genetic disorder caused by **partial deletions of mitochondrial DNA (delta-mtDNA)** and **duplication of mitochondrial DNA (dup-mtDNA)**. The partial deletions of mtDNA have been associated with a marked reduction in the enzymatic activity of NADH dehydrogenase (complex I), succinate dehydrogenase (complex II), ubiquinone-cytochrome c oxidoreductase (complex III), and cytochrome oxidase (complex IV).
2. Heteroplasmy is common, and expression of the disease is highly variable.
3. **Clinical features include**: chronic progressive external ophthalmoplegia (CPEO; degeneration of the motor nerves of the eye), pigmentary degeneration of the retina ("salt and pepper" appearance), heart block, short stature, gonadal failure, diabetes mellitus, thyroid disease, deafness, vestibular dysfunction, cerebellar ataxia, and onset occurring at ≈20 years of age.

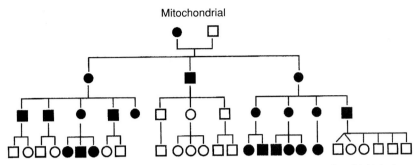

● **Figure 8-1 Pedigree of mitochondrial inheritance.** Typical pedigree seen in mitochondrial inheritance. Inheritance is matrilineal, with all children of affected mothers being affected but not children of affected fathers. Affected fathers do not produce affected children.

TABLE 8-1	GENETIC DISORDERS INVOLVING MITOCHONDRIA	
Genetic Disorder	**Gene/Gene Product**	**Clinical Features**
LHON	*ND4* gene/subunit 4 of NADH dehydrogenase *ND1* gene/subunit 1 of NADH dehydrogenase *ND6* gene/subunit 6 of NADH dehydrogenase	Progressive optic nerve degeneration that results clinically in blindness, blurred vision, or loss of central vision; telangiectatic microangiopathy; disk pseudoedema; vascular tortuosity; onset occurring at ≈20 years of age with precipitous vision loss; and males affected far more often than females for some unknown reason.
MERRF	*tRNA^{Lys}* gene NADH dehydrogenase (complex I) and cytochrome oxidase (complex IV) are affected.	Myoclonus (muscle twitching), seizures, cerebellar ataxia, dementia, mitochondrial myopathy (abnormal mitochondria within skeletal muscle that impart an irregular shape and blotchy red appearance to the muscle cells, hence the term *ragged red fibers*)
MELAS	*tRNA^{Leu}* gene Cytochrome oxidase (complex IV) is affected.	Mitochondrial myopathy, encephalopathy, lactic acidosis, and strokelike episodes
Kearns-Sayre syndrome	Delta-mtDNA Dup-mtDNA NADH dehydrogenase (complex I), succinate dehydrogenase (complex II), ubiquinone-cytochrome c oxidoreductase (complex III), and cytochrome oxidase (complex IV) are affected.	CPEO (degeneration of the motor nerves of the eye), pigmentary degeneration of the retina ("salt and pepper" appearance), heart block, short stature, gonadal failure, diabetes mellitus, thyroid disease, deafness, vestibular dysfunction, cerebellar ataxia, and onset occurring at ≈20 years of age

LHON, Leber hereditary optic neuropathy; MERRF, myoclonic epilepsy with ragged red fibers syndrome; NADH, nicotinamide adenine dinucleotide; MELAS, mitochondrial myopathy, encephalopathy, lactic acidosis, strokelike episodes syndrome; CPEO, chronic progressive external ophthalmoplegia.

Chapter 9
Mitosis, Meiosis, and Gametogenesis

1 Mitosis (Figure 9-1). Mitosis is the process that occurs when a cell with the diploid number of chromosomes, which in humans is 46, passes on the diploid number of chromosomes to daughter cells. The term *diploid* is classically used to refer to a cell containing 46 chromosomes. The term *haploid* is classically used to refer to a cell containing 23 chromosomes. The process ensures that the diploid number of 46 chromosomes is maintained in the cells. Mitosis occurs at the end of a cell cycle. Phases of the cell cycle include the following:

A. **G_0 (GAP) PHASE.** The G_0 phase is the resting phase of the cell. The amount of time a cell spends in G_0 is variable and depends on how actively a cell is dividing.

B. **G_1 PHASE.** The G_1 phase is the gap of time between mitosis (M phase) and DNA synthesis (S phase). The G_1 phase is the phase where **RNA, protein, and organelle synthesis** occurs. The G_1 phase lasts about **5 hours** in a typical mammalian cell with a 16-hour cell cycle.

C. **G_1 CHECKPOINT.** **Cdk2-cyclin D and Cdk2-cyclin E** mediate the **$G_1 \rightarrow$ S phase** transition at the G_1 checkpoint.

D. **S (SYNTHESIS) PHASE.** The S phase is the phase where **DNA synthesis** occurs. The S phase lasts about **7 hours** in a typical mammalian cell with a 16-hour cell cycle.

E. **G_2 PHASE.** The G_2 phase is the gap of time between DNA synthesis (S phase) and mitosis (M phase). The G_2 phase is the phase where high levels of **ATP synthesis** occur. The G_2 phase lasts about **3 hours** in a typical mammalian cell with a 16-hour cell cycle.

F. **G_2 CHECKPOINT.** **Cdk1-cyclin A and Cdk1-cyclin B** mediate the **$G_2 \rightarrow$ M phase** transition at the G_2 checkpoint.

G. **M (MITOSIS) PHASE.** The M phase is the phase where **cell division** occurs. The M phase is divided into six stages called *prophase, prometaphase, metaphase, anaphase, telophase,* and *cytokinesis*. The M phase lasts about 1 hour in a typical mammalian cell with a 16-hour cell cycle.
   1. **Prophase.** The chromatin condenses to form well-defined chromosomes. Each chromosome has been duplicated during the S phase and has a specific DNA sequence called the *centromere* that is required for proper segregation. The **centrosome complex**, which is the **microtubule organizing center (MTOC)**, splits into two, and each half begins to move to opposite poles of the cell. The **mitotic spindle** (microtubules) forms between the centrosomes.
   2. **Prometaphase.** The nuclear envelope is disrupted, which allows the microtubules access to the chromosomes. The nucleolus disappears. The **kinetochores** (protein

complexes) assemble at each centromere on the chromosomes. Certain micro-tubules of the mitotic spindle bind to the kinetochores and are called *kinetochore microtubules*. Other microtubules of the mitotic spindle are now called *polar microtubules* and *astral microtubules*.

3. **Metaphase.** The chromosomes align at the metaphase plate. The cells can be arrested in this stage by microtubule inhibitors (e.g., colchicine). Cells arrested in this stage can be used for **karyotype analysis.**

4. **Anaphase.** The centromeres split, kinetochores separate, and chromosomes move to opposite poles. The kinetochore microtubules shorten. The polar microtubules lengthen.

5. **Telophase.** The chromosomes begin to decondense to form chromatin. The nuclear envelope re-forms. The nucleolus reappears. The kinetochore micro-tubules disappear. The polar microtubules continue to lengthen.

6. **Cytokinesis.** The cytoplasm divides by a process called *cleavage*. A **cleavage fur-row** forms around the middle of the cell. A **contractile ring** consisting of actin and myosin filaments is found at the cleavage furrow.

Ⅱ Checkpoints

A. The checkpoints in the cell cycle **are** specialized signaling mechanisms that regulate and coordinate the cell response to **DNA damage** and **replication fork blockage.** When the extent of DNA damage or replication fork blockage is beyond the steady-state threshold of DNA repair pathways, a checkpoint signal is produced and a checkpoint is activated. The activation of a checkpoint slows down the cell cycle so that DNA repair may occur and/or blocked replication forks can be recovered.

B. The two main protein families that control the cell cycle are **cyclins and** the **cyclin-dependent protein kinases (Cdks).** A cyclin is a protein that regulates the activity of Cdks and are named because cyclins undergo a cycle of synthesis and degradation dur-ing the cell cycle. The cyclins and Cdks form complexes called *Cdk-cyclin complexes*. The ability of Cdks to phosphorylate target proteins is dependent on the particular cyclin that complexes with it.

Ⅲ Meiosis (Figure 9-2).
Meiosis is the process of **germ cell division** (contrasted with mitosis, which is **somatic cell division**) that occurs only in the production of the germ cells (i.e., sperm in the testes and oocyte in the ovary). In general, meiosis consists of two cell divisions (meiosis I and meiosis II) but only one round of DNA replication that results in the formation of four gametes, each containing half the number of chromosomes (23 chro-mosomes) and half the amount of DNA (1N) found in normal somatic cells (46 chromo-somes, 2N). The various aspects of meiosis compared with mitosis are given in Table 9-1.

A. MEIOSIS I. Events that occur during meiosis I include the following:
1. **DNA replication.**
2. **Synapsis.** Synapsis refers to the pairing of each duplicated chromosome with its homologue, which occurs only in meiosis I (not meiosis II or mitosis).
   a. In female meiosis, each chromosome has a homologous partner, so the two X chromosomes synapse and cross over just like the other pairs of homologous chromosomes.
   b. In male meiosis, there is a problem because the X and Y chromosomes are very different. However, the X and Y chromosomes do pair and cross over. The

pairing of the X and Y chromosomes is in an **end-to-end fashion** (rather than along the whole length as for all other chromosomes), which is made possible by a 2.6 Mb region of sequence homology between the X and Y chromosomes at the tips of their p arms where crossover occurs. This region of homology is called the *pseudoautosomal region*.

c. Although the X and Y chromosomes are not homologs, they are functionally homologous in meiosis, so there are 23 homologous pairs of the 46 duplicated chromosomes in the cell at this point.

3. **Crossover.** Crossover refers to the **equal exchange** of large segments of DNA between the maternal chromatid and paternal chromatid (i.e., nonsister chromatids) at the **chiasma**, which occurs during prophase (pachytene stage) of meiosis I. Chiasma is the location where crossover occurs forming a X-shaped chromosome and named for the Greek letter *chi*, which is X-shaped also.

a. Crossover introduces **one level of genetic variability** among the gametes.

b. During crossover, two other events (i.e., **unequal crossover** and **unequal sister chromatid exchange**) may occur, which introduces **variable number tandem repeat (VNTR) polymorphisms, duplications, or deletions** into the human nuclear genome.

4. **Alignment.** Alignment refers to the process whereby homologous duplicated chromosomes align at the metaphase plate. At this stage, there are still 23 pairs of the 46 chromosomes in the cell.

5. **Disjunction.** Disjunction refers to the separation of the 46 maternal and paternal duplicated chromosomes in the 23 homologous pairs from each other into separate secondary gametocytes (*Note:* the **centromeres do not split**).

a. The choice of which maternal or paternal homologous duplicated chromosomes enter the secondary gametocyte is a **random distribution**.

b. There are 2^{23} (**or 8.4 million**) possible ways that the maternal and paternal homologous duplicated chromosomes can be combined. This random distribution of maternal and paternal homologous duplicated chromosomes introduces **another level of genetic variability** among the gametes.

6. **Cell division.** Meiosis I is often called the *reduction division*, because the number of chromosomes is reduced by half, to the haploid (23 duplicated chromosomes, 2N DNA content) number in the two secondary gametocytes that are formed.

B. **MEIOSIS II.** Events that occur during meiosis II include:

1. **Synapsis:** Absent.

2. **Crossover:** Absent.

3. **Alignment:** 23 duplicated chromosomes align at the metaphase plate.

4. **Disjunction:** 23 duplicated chromosomes separate to form 23 single chromosomes when the **centromeres split**.

5. **Cell division:** gametes (23 single chromosomes, 1N) are formed.

Ⅳ Oogenesis: Female Gametogenesis

A. **Primordial germ cells (46,2N)** from the wall of the yolk sac arrive in the ovary at **week 4** and differentiate into **oogonia (46,2N)**, which populate the ovary through <u>mitotic</u> division.

B. Oogonia enter meiosis I and undergo DNA replication to form **primary oocytes (46,4N)**. All primary oocytes are formed by the **month 5 of fetal life.** No oogonia are present at birth. Primary oocytes remain **dormant in prophase (diplotene) of meiosis I** from month 5 of fetal life until puberty at $\approx$12 years of age (or ovulation at $\approx$50 years of age given that some primary oocytes will remain dormant until menopause).

C. After puberty, 5–15 primary oocytes will begin maturation with each ovarian cycle, with usually only one reaching full maturity in each cycle.

D. During the ovarian cycle, a primary oocyte completes meiosis I to form two daughter cells: the **secondary oocyte (23 chromosomes, 2N amount of DNA)** and the **first polar body** that degenerates.

E. The secondary oocyte promptly begins meiosis II but is **arrested in metaphase of meiosis II** about 3 hours before ovulation. The secondary oocyte remains arrested in the metaphase of meiosis II until fertilization occurs.

F. At fertilization, the secondary oocyte will complete meiosis II to form **one mature oocyte (23,1N)** and a **second polar body.**

Ⅴ Spermatogenesis. Male gametogenesis is classically divided into three phases:

A. SPERMATOCYTOGENESIS. Primordial germ cells (46,2N) form the wall of the yolk sac, arrive in the testes at **week 4,** and remain **dormant until puberty.** At puberty, primordial germ cells differentiate into **type A spermatogonia (46,2N).** Type A spermatogonia undergo mitosis to provide a continuous supply of stem cells throughout the reproductive life of the male. Some type A spermatogonia differentiate into **type B spermatogonia (46,2N).**

B. MEIOSIS. Type B spermatogonia enter meiosis I and undergo DNA replication to form **primary spermatocytes (46,4N).** Primary spermatocytes complete meiosis I to form **secondary spermatocytes (23,2N).** Secondary spermatocytes complete meiosis II to form **four spermatids (23,1N).**

C. SPERMIOGENESIS. Spermatids undergo a **post-meiotic series of morphologic changes** to form **sperm (23,1N).** These changes include: formation of the acrosome; condensation of the nucleus; and formation of head, neck, and tail.
1. The total time of sperm formation (from spermatogonia to spermatozoa) is about 64 days.
2. Newly ejaculated sperm are incapable of fertilization until they undergo **capacitation,** which occurs in the female reproductive tract and involves the unmasking of sperm glycosyltransferases and removal of proteins coating the surface of the sperm. Capacitation occurs before the acrosome reaction.

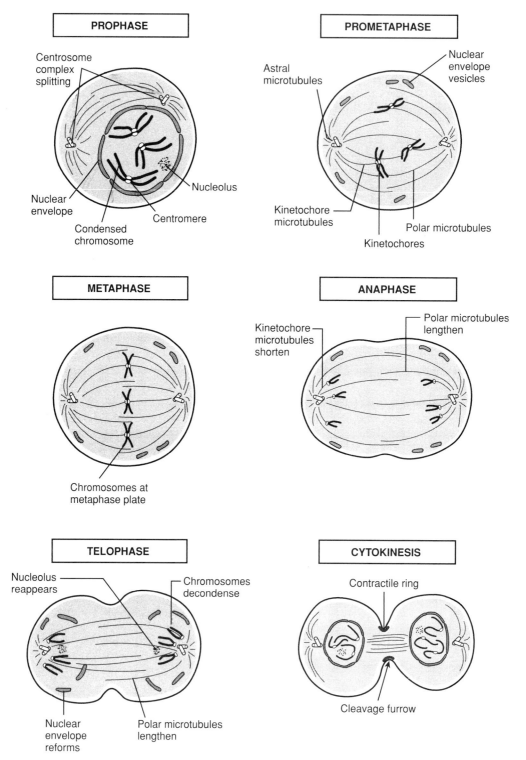

● **Figure 9-1 Diagram of the stages of the M (mitosis) phase.** For the sake of simplicity, only 3 chromosomes (out of the 46 chromosomes in a human cell) are represented.

A

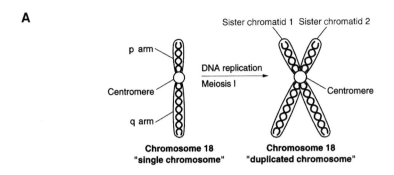

B

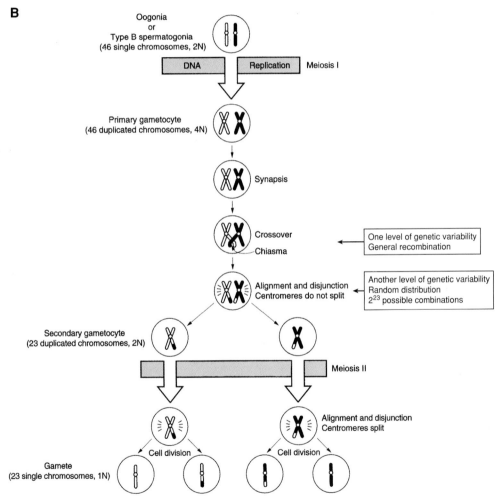

● **Figure 9-2 Meiosis. A:** Schematic diagram of chromosome 18 shown in its "single chromosome" state and "dupli-cated chromosome" state that is formed by DNA replication during meiosis I. It is important to understand that both the single chromosome state and duplicated chromosome state will be counted as one chromosome 18. As long as the additional DNA in the duplicated chromosome is bound at the centromere, the structure will be counted as one chromosome 18 even though it has twice the amount of DNA. The duplicated chromosome is often referred to as consisting of two sister chromatids (chromatid 1 and chromatid 2). **B:** Schematic representation of meiosis I and meiosis II, emphasizing the changes in chromosome number and amount of DNA that occur during gametogenesis. Only one pair of homologous chromosomes is shown. (White, maternal origin; black, paternal origin.) The point at which DNA crosses over is called the *chiasma*. Segments of DNA are exchanged, thereby introducing genetic variability to the gametes. In addition, various cell types along with their appropriate designation of number of chromosomes and amount of DNA is shown.

TABLE 9-1	COMPARISON OF MEIOSIS AND MITOSIS
Meiosis	**Mitosis**
Occurs only in the testis and ovary	Occurs in a wide variety of tissues and organs
Produces haploid (23,1N) gametes (sperm and secondary oocyte)	Produces diploid (46,2N) somatic daughter cells
Involves two cell divisions and one round of DNA replication	Involves one cell division and one round of DNA replication
Stages of Meiosis	**Stages of Mitosis**
Meiosis I	***Interphase***
Prophase	G_0 phase
Leptotene (long, thin DNA strands)	G_1 phase
Zygotene (synapsis occurs; synaptonemal complex)	G_1 checkpoint
Pachytene (crossover occurs; short, thick DNA strands)	S phase
Diplotene (chromosomes separate except at centromere)	G_2 phase G_2 checkpoint
Prometaphase	***Mitosis phase***
Metaphase	Prophase
Anaphase	Prometaphase
Telophase	Metaphase
Meiosis II (essentially identical to mitosis)	Anaphase
Prophase	Telophase
Prometaphase	
Metaphase	
Anaphase	
Telophase	
Male: Prophase of meiosis I lasts ≈22 days and completes meiosis II in a few hours	Interphase lasts ≈15 hours
Female: Prophase of meiosis I lasts from ≈12 (puberty) to 50 years of age (menopause) and completes meiosis II when fertilization occurs	M phase lasts ≈1 hour
Pairing of homologous chromosomes occurs.	There is no pairing of homologous chromosomes.
Genetic recombination occurs (exchange of large segments of maternal and paternal DNA via crossover during meiosis I).	Genetic recombination does not occur.
Maternal and paternal homologous chromosomes are randomly distributed among the gametes to ensure genetic variability.	Maternal and paternal homologous chromosomes are faithfully distributed among the daughter cells to ensure genetic similarity.
Gametes are genetically different.	Daughter cells are genetically identical.

Chapter **10**

Chromosome Morphology Methods

I **Studying Human Chromosomes.** Mitotic chromosomes are fairly easy to study because they can be observed in any cell undergoing mitosis. Meiotic chromosomes are much more difficult to study because they can be observed only in ovarian or testicular samples. In the female, meiosis is especially difficult because meiosis occurs during fetal development. In the male, meiotic chromosomes can be studied only in a testicular biopsy of an adult male. Any tissue that can be grown in culture can be used for **karyotype analysis**, but only certain tissue samples are suitable for some kinds of studies. For example, chorionic villi or amniocytes from amniotic fluid are used for prenatal studies; bone marrow is usually the most appropriate tissue for leukemia studies; skin or placenta is used for miscarriage studies; and blood for patients with dysmorphic features, unexplained mental retardation, or any other suspected genetic conditions. Whatever the tissue used, the cells must be grown in tissue culture for some period of time until optimal growth occurs. Blood cells must have a mitogen added to the culture media to stimulate the **mitosis** of lympocytes, but other tissues can be grown without such stimulation.

A. Once a tissue has reached its optimal time for a harvest, **colchicine** (colcemid) is added to the media, which arrests the cells in **metaphase**.

B. The cells are then concentrated, treated with a hypotonic solution that aids in the spreading of the chromosomes, and finally fixed with an acetic acid/methanol solution.

C. The cell preparation is then dropped onto microscope slides and stained by a variety of methods (see below).

D. It is often preferable to use **prometaphase** chromosomes in cytogenetic analysis, as they are less condensed and therefore show more detail. In cytogenetic analysis, separated prometaphase or metaphase chromosomes are identified and photographed or digitized.

E. The chromosomes in the photograph of the metaphase are then cut out and arranged in a standard pattern called the *karyotype* or, in the case of digital images, arranged into a karyotype with the assistance of a computer.

II **Staining of Chromosomes.** Metaphase or prometaphase chromosomes may be prepared for karyotype analysis and then stained by various techniques. In addition, one of the great advantages of some staining techniques is that metaphase or prometaphase chromosomes are not required.

A. CHROMOSOME BANDING. Chromosome banding techniques are based on denaturation and/or enzymatic digestion of DNA followed by incorporation of a DNA-binding dye. This results in chromosomes staining as a series of dark and light bands.

1. **G-Banding.** G-banding uses trypsin denaturation before staining with the Giemsa dye and is now the standard analytical method in cytogenetics.
   a. Giemsa staining produces a unique pattern of **dark bands** (**Giemsa positive; G bands**) that consist of heterochromatin, replicate in the late S phase, are rich in A-T bases, and contain few genes.
   b. Giemsa staining also produces a unique pattern of **light bands** (**Giemsa negative; R bands**) that consist of euchromatin, replicate in the early S phase, are rich in G-C bases, and contain many genes.
2. **R-Banding.** R-banding uses the Giemsa dye (as above) to visualize **light bands** (**Giemsa negative; R bands**) that essentially are the reverse of the G-banding pattern. R-banding can also be visualized by G-C specific dyes (e.g., chromomycin A_3, oligomycin, or mithramycin).
3. **Q-Banding.** Q-banding uses the fluorochrome quinacrine (binds preferentially to A-T bases) to visualize **Q bands**, which essentially are the same as G bands.
4. **T-Banding.** T-banding uses severe heat denaturation prior to Giemsa staining or a combination of dyes and fluorochromes to visualize **T bands**, which are a subset of R bands located at the telomeres.
5. **C-Banding.** C-banding uses barium hydroxide denaturation prior to Giemsa staining to visualize **C bands**, which are constitutive heterochromatin located mainly at the centromere.

B. **FLUORESCENCE IN SITU HYBRIDIZATION (FISH).** The FISH technique is based on the ability of single-stranded DNA (i.e., a DNA probe) to hybridize (bind or anneal) to its complementary target sequence on a unique DNA sequence that the clinician is interested in localizing on the chromosome. Once this unique DNA sequence is known, a fluorescent DNA probe can be constructed. The fluorescent DNA probe is allowed to hybridize with chromosomes prepared for karyotype analysis and thereby visualize the unique DNA sequence on specific chromosomes.

C. **CHROMOSOME PAINTING.** The chromosome painting technique is based on the construction of fluorescent DNA probes to a wide variety of different DNA fragments from a single chromosome. The fluorescent DNA probes are allowed to hybridize with chromosomes prepared for karyotype analysis and thereby visualize many different loci spanning one whole chromosome (i.e., a chromosome paint). Essentially, one whole particular chromosome will fluoresce.

D. **SPECTRAL KARYOTYPING OR 24 COLOR CHROMOSOME PAINTING.** The spectral karyotyping technique is based on chromosome painting, whereby DNA probes for all 24 chromosomes are labeled with five different fluorochromes so that each of the 24 chromosomes will have a different ratio of fluorochromes. The different fluorochrome ratios cannot be detected by the naked eye, but computer software can analyze the different ratios and assign a pseudocolor for each ratio. This allows all 24 chromosomes to be painted with a different color. Essentially, all 24 chromosomes will be painted a different color. The homologues of each chromosome will be painted the same color, but the X and Y chromosomes will be different colors, so 24 different colors are required.

E. **COMPARATIVE GENOME HYBRIDIZATION (CGH).** The CGH technique is based on the competitive hybridization of two fluorescent DNA probes: one DNA probe from a normal cell labeled with a red fluorochrome and the other DNA probe from a tumor cell labeled with a green fluorochrome. The fluorescent DNA probes are mixed together and allowed to hybridize with chromosomes prepared for karyotype analysis. The ratio of red-to-green signal is plotted along the length of each chromosome as a distribution line. The red-to-green ratio should be 1:1 unless the tumor DNA is missing some of the chromosomal regions present in normal DNA (more red fluorochrome and the distribution line shifts to the left) or the tumor DNA has more of some chromosomal regions than present in normal DNA (more green fluorochrome and the distribution line shifts to the right).

III Chromosome Appearance (Figure 10-1)

A. The appearance of chromosomal DNA can vary considerably in a normal resting cell (e.g., degree of packaging, euchromatin, heterochromatin) and a dividing cell (e.g., mitosis and meiosis). It is important to note that the pictures of chromosomes seen in karyotype analysis are chromosomal DNA at a particular point in time (i.e., arrested at the metaphase [or prometaphase] of mitosis).

B. Early metaphase karyograms showed chromosomes as X-shaped because the chromosomes were at a point in mitosis when the protein **cohesin** no longer bound the sister chromatids together but the centromeres had not yet separated.

C. Modern metaphase karyograms show chromosomes as I-shaped because the chromosomes are at a point in mitosis when the protein cohesin still binds the sister chromatids together and the centromeres are not separated. In addition, many modern karyograms are prometaphase karyograms, where the chromosomes are I-shaped.

IV Chromosome Nomenclature

A. A chromosome consists of two characteristic parts called *arms*. The short arm is called the *p (petit) arm*, and the long arm is called the *q (queue) arm*.

B. The arms of G-banded and R-banded chromosomes can be subdivided into **regions** (counting outward from the centromere), **subregions (bands)**, **sub-bands** (noted by the addition of a decimal point), and **sub-sub bands**.

C. For example, 6p21.34 is read as the short arm of chromosome 6, region 2, subregion (band) 1, sub-band 3, and sub-sub band 4. This is **NOT** read as the short arm of chromosome 6, twenty-one point thirty-four.

D. In addition, locations on an arm can be referred to in anatomical terms: **proximal** is closer to the centromere, and **distal** is farther from the centromere.

E. The chromosome banding patterns of human G-banded chromosomes have been standardized and are represented diagrammatically in an idiogram.

F. A **metacentric chromosome** refers to a chromosome where the centromere is close to the midpoint, thereby dividing the chromosome into roughly equal length arms.

G. A **submetacentric chromosome** refers to a chromosome where the centromere is far away from the midpoint so that a p arm and q arm can be distinguished.

H. A **telocentric chromosome** refers to a chromosome where the centromere is at the very end of the chromosome so that only the q arm is described.

I. An **acrocentric chromosome** refers to a chromosome where the centromere is near the end of the chromosome so that the p arm is very short (just discernible).

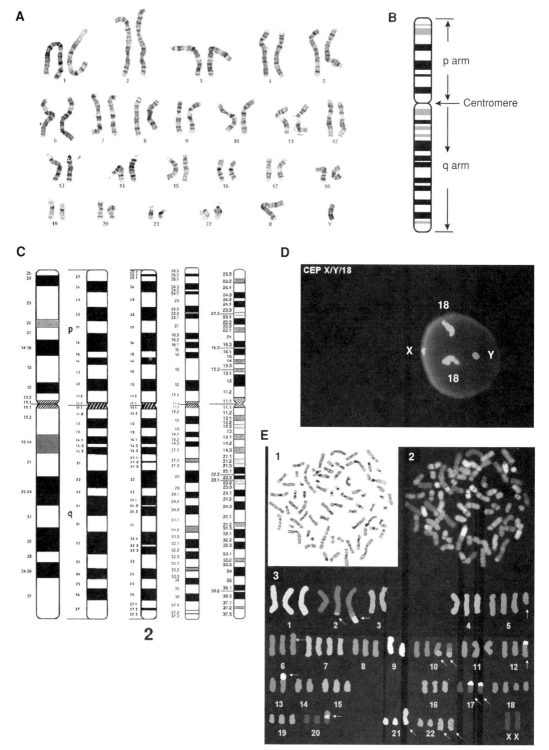

● Figure 10-1 **Karyotypes and chromosome morphology. A:** G-banded metaphase chromosomes arranged in a karyotype. **B:** Diagram of a metaphase chromosome showing the centromere, p arm, and q arm. **C:** Chromosome 2 is shown (from left to right) at different levels of resolution starting with approximately 300 bands and proceeding to 400-, 550-, 700-, and 850 band levels. **D:** FISH for sex determination. Note the one X chromosome and the one Y chromosome, indicating a male. Chromosome 18 is the autosomal control. **E:** Spectral karyotyping of a chronic myelogenous leukemia cell line demonstrating a complex karyotype with several structural and numeric chromosome aberrations. **E1:** A metaphase cell showing the G- banding pattern. **E2:** The same metaphase cell as in E1 showing the spectral display pattern. **E3:** The same metaphase cell as in E1 and E2 arranged as a karyotype. *Arrows* indicate structural chromosome aberrations involving two or more different chromosomes.

Chapter 11

Cytogenetic Disorders

Ⅰ Numerical Chromosomal Anomalies

A. **Polyploidy** is the addition of an extra haploid set or sets of chromosomes (i.e., 23) to the normal diploid set of chromosomes (i.e., 46).

   1. **Triploidy** is a condition whereby cells contain **69 chromosomes.**

     a. Triploidy occurs as a result of either a **failure of meiosis in a germ cell** (e.g., fertilization of a diploid egg by a haploid sperm) or **dispermy** (two sperm that fertilize one egg).

     b. Triploidy results in spontaneous abortion of the conceptus or brief survival of the live-born infant after birth.

   2. **Tetraploidy** is a condition whereby cells contain **92 chromosomes.**

     a. Tetraploidy occurs as a result of **failure of the first cleavage division.**

     b. Tetraploidy almost always results in spontaneous abortion of the conceptus with survival to birth being an extremely rare occurrence.

B. **Aneuploidy (Figure 11-1)** is the addition of one chromosome (**trisomy**), or loss of one chromosome (**monosomy**). Aneuploidy occurs as a result of **nondisjunction during meiosis.**

   1. **Trisomy 21 (Down syndrome).**

     a. Down syndrome is a trisomic condition linked to a specific region on chromosome 21 called the *Down syndrome critical region.* Down syndrome may also be caused by a specific type of translocation, called a *Robertsonian translocation,* that occurs between acrocentric chromosomes.

     b. Trisomy 21 frequency increases with **advanced maternal age.** The triple marker for Down syndrome includes **low α-fetoprotein levels (↓AFP)** in amniotic fluid or maternal serum; **high human chorionic gonadotropin (↑hCG)** in amniotic fluid or maternal serum; and **low unconjugated estriol (↓estriol)** in urine.

     c. **Clinical features include:** moderate mental retardation (the leading type of mental retardation), microcephaly, microphthalmia, colobomata, cataracts and glaucoma, flat nasal bridge, epicanthal folds, protruding tongue, simian crease in hand, increased nuchal skin folds, appearance of an "X" across the face when the baby cries, and congenital heart defects. Alzheimer neurofibrillary tangles and plaques are found in Down syndrome patients over 30 years of age. A condition mimicking acute megakaryocytic leukemia frequently occurs in children with Down syndrome, and they are at increased risk for developing acute lymphoblastic leukemia.

   2. **Klinefelter syndrome (47,XXY).**

     a. Klinefelter syndrome is a **trisomic** sex chromosome condition **found only in males.**

b.   **Clinical features include**: varicose veins, arterial and venous leg ulcer, scant body and pubic hair, male hypogonadism, sterility with fibrosis of seminiferous tubules, marked decrease in testosterone levels, elevated gonadotropin levels, gynecomastia, IQ slightly less than that of siblings, learning disabilities, antisocial behavior, delayed speech as a child, tall stature, and eunuchoid habitus.

3.   Turner syndrome (monosomy X; usually 45, X but can be mosaic).
a.   Turner syndrome is a monosomic condition **found only in females.**
b.   **Clinical features include**: short stature, low-set ears, ocular hypertelorism, ptosis, low posterior hairline, webbed neck due to a remnant of a fetal cystic hygroma, congenital hypoplasia of lymphatics causing peripheral edema of hands and feet, shield chest, pinpoint nipples, congenital heart defects, aortic coarctation, female hypogonadism, ovarian fibrous streaks (i.e., infertility), primary amenorrhea, and absence of secondary sex characteristics.

C.   Mixoploidy is a condition where a person has two or more genetically different cell populations. If the genetically different cell populations arise from a single zygote, the condition is called *mosaicism*. If the genetically different cell populations arise from different zygotes, the condition is called *chimerism*.

1.   Mosaicism.
a.   A person may become a mosaic by **post-zygotic mutations** that can occur at any time during postzygotic life.
b.   These post-zygotic mutations are actually quite frequent in humans and produce genetically different cell populations (i.e., most of us are mosaics to a certain extent). However, these post-zygotic mutations usually are not clinically significant.
c.   If the post-zygotic mutation produces a substantial clone of mutated cells, then a clinical consequence may occur.
d.   The formation of a substantial clone of mutated cells can occur in two ways: the mutation results in an abnormal proliferation of cells (e.g., formation of cancer) or the mutation occurs in a progenitor cell during early embryonic life and forms a significant clone of mutated cells.
e.   A post-zygotic mutation may also cause a clinical consequence if the mutation occurs in the germ line cells of a parent (called *germinal* or *gonadal mosaicism*). For example, if a post-zygotic mutation occurs in male spermatogenic cells, then the man may harbor a large clone of mutant sperm without any clinical consequence (i.e., the man is normal). However, if the mutant sperm from the normal male fertilizes a secondary oocyte, the infant may have a *de novo* inherited disease. This means that a normal couple without any history of inherited disease may have a child with a *de novo* inherited disease if one of the parents is a gonadal mosaic.

2.   Chimerism. A person may become a chimera by the fusion of two genetically different zygotes to form a single embryo (i.e., the reverse of twinning) or by the limited colonization of one twin by cells from a genetically different (i.e., nonidentical, fraternal) cotwin.

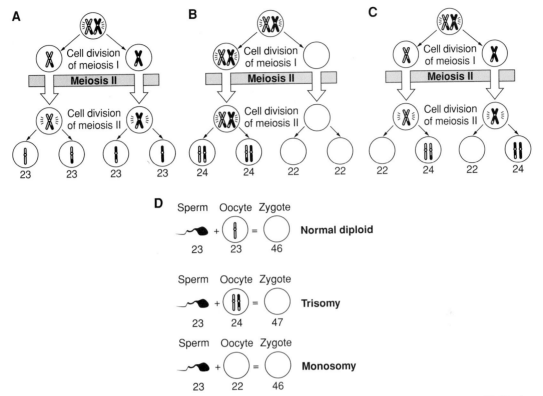

● **Figure 11-1 Meiosis and nondisjunction. A:** Normal meiotic divisions (I and II) producing gametes with 23 chromosomes. **B:** Nondisjunction occurring in meiosis I producing gametes with 24 and 22 chromosomes. **C:** Nondisjunction occurring in meiosis II producing gametes with 24 and 22 chromosomes. **D:** Although nondisjunction may occur in either spermatogenesis or oogenesis, there is a higher frequency of nondisjunction in oogenesis. In this schematic, nondisjunction in oogenesis is depicted. If an abnormal oocyte (24 chromosomes) is fertilized by a normal sperm (23 chromosomes), a zygote with 47 chromosomes is produced (i.e., trisomy). If an abnormal oocyte (22 chromosomes) is fertilized by a normal sperm (23 chromosomes), a zygote with 45 chromosomes is produced (i.e., monosomy).

Ⅱ   Structural Chromosomal Abnormalities

A. **Deletions** are a loss of chromatin from a chromosome. There is much variability in the clinical presentations based on the particular genes and the number of genes that are deleted. Some of the more common deletion abnormalities are indicated below.

    1. **Chromosome 4p deletion (Wolf-Hirschhorn syndrome).**

        a. Wolf-Hirschhorn syndrome is caused by a deletion in the short arm of **chromosome 4 (4p16).**

        b. **Clinical features include:** prominent forehead and broad nasal root ("Greek warrior helmet"), short philtrum, down-turned mouth, congenital heart defects, growth retardation, and severe mental retardation.

    2. **Chromosome 5p deletion (Cri-du-chat ["cat cry"] syndrome).**

        a. Cri-du-chat syndrome is caused by a deletion in the short arm of **chromosome 5 (5p15).**

        b. **Clinical features include:** round facies, a catlike cry, congenital heart defects, microcephaly, and mental retardation.

B. Microdeletions are a loss of chromatin from a chromosome that cannot be detected easily, even by high-resolution banding. Fluorescence in situ hybridization (FISH) is the definitive test for detecting microdeletions.

1. **Prader-Willi syndrome (PW).**
   a. PW is caused by a microdeletion in the long arm of **chromosome 15 (15q11.2-13)** derived from the **father**.
   b. PW illustrates the phenomenon of **genomic imprinting**, which is the differential expression of genes depending on the parent of origin. The mechanism of inactivation (or genomic imprinting) involves **DNA methylation of cytosine nucleotides** during gametogenesis resulting in transcriptional inactivation.
   c. The counterpart of PW is **Angelman syndrome**. Other examples that highlight the role of genomic imprinting include **hydatidiform moles** and **Beckwith-Wiedemann syndrome (BWS)**. BWS is associated with a number of candidate genes (e.g., growth factor and tumor suppressor genes) on the chromosome 11p15 region and has the following clinical features: macrosomia, macroglossia, visceromegaly, embryonal tumors (e.g., Wilms tumor, hepatoblastoma, neuroblastoma, rhabdomyosarcoma), omphalocele, neonatal hypoglycemia, ear creases/pits, adrenocortical cytomegaly, and renal abnormalities.
   d. **Clinical features include**: poor feeding and hypotonia at birth followed by hyperphagia (insatiable appetite), hypogonadism, obesity, short stature, small hands and feet, behavior problems (rage, violence), and mild to moderate mental retardation.

2. **Angelman syndrome (AS; happy puppet syndrome).**
   a. AS is caused by a microdeletion in the long arm of **chromosome 15 (15q11.2-13)** derived from the **mother**.
   b. AS is an example of **genomic imprinting** (see above). The counterpart of AS is **Prader-Willi syndrome**.
   c. **Clinical features include**: gait ataxia (stiff, jerky, unsteady, upheld arms), seizures, happy disposition with inappropriate laughter, and severe mental retardation (only 5–10-word vocabulary).

3. **DiGeorge syndrome (DS; catch-22; 22q11 syndrome).**
   a. DS is caused by a microdeletion in the long arm of **chromosome 22 (22q11.2)**, which is also called the *DiGeorge chromosomal region*.
   b. DS occurs when **pharyngeal pouches 3 and 4** fail to differentiate into the thymus and parathyroid glands.
   c. DS has a phenotypic and genotypic similarity to **velocardiofacial syndrome (VCFS)**, that is, both DS and VCFS are manifestations of a microdeletion at 22q11.2.
   d. **Clinical features include**: facial anomalies resembling first arch syndrome (micrognathia, low-set ears) due to abnormal neural crest cell migration, cardiovascular anomalies due to abnormal neural crest cell migration during formation of the aorticopulmonary septum, immunodeficiency due to absence of the thymus gland, and hypocalcemia due to absence of parathyroid glands.

4. **WAGR syndrome.**
   a. WAGR is caused by a microdeletion in the short arm of **chromosome 11p13** where the *WT1* gene (Wilms tumor gene 1) is located.
   b. The *WT1* gene encodes for a zinc finger DNA-binding protein that is required by normal embryologic development of the genitourinary system. *WT1* gene isoforms synergize with steroidogenic factor-1 **(SF-1)**, which is a nuclear receptor that regulates the transcription of a number of genes involved in reproduction, steroidogenesis, and male sexual development.

      c.   **Clinical features include**: Wilms tumor, aniridia (absence of the iris), genitourinary abnormalities (e.g., gonadoblastoma), and mental retardation.

C. **Translocations (Figure 11-2)** result from breakage and exchange of segments between chromosomes.

    1. **Robertsonian translocation (RT).**

        a.   RT is caused by translocations between the long arms (q) of acrocentric (satellite) chromosomes where the breakpoint is near the centromere. The short arms (p) of these chromosomes are generally lost.

        b.   Carriers of RT are **clinically normal** since the short arms, which are lost, contain only inert DNA and some rRNA (ribosomal RNA) genes, which occur in multiple copies on other chromosomes.

        c.   One of the most common translocations found in humans is **RT t(14q21q).**

        d.   The clinical issue in RT t(14q21q) occurs when the carriers produce gametes by meiosis and reproduce. Depending on how the chromosomes segregate during meiosis, conception can produce offspring with translocation trisomy 21 (live birth), translocation trisomy 14 (early miscarriage), monosomy 14 or 21 (early miscarriage), a normal chromosome complement (live birth), or a t(14q21q) carrier (live birth).

        e.   A couple where one member is a t(14q21q) carrier may have a baby with translocation trisomy 21 (Down syndrome) or recurrent miscarriages.

    2. **Reciprocal translocation (RC).**

        a.   RC is caused by the exchange of segments between two chromosomes that forms two derivative (der) chromosomes with each containing a segment of the other chromosome from the reciprocal exchange.

        b.   One of the most common inherited RCs found in humans is the t(11;22)(q23.3;q11.2).

        c.   The translocation heterozygote, or carrier, would be at risk of having a child with abnormalities due to passing on only one of the derivative chromosomes. That would result in a child who would be partially trisomic for one of the participant chromosomes and partially monosomic for the other.

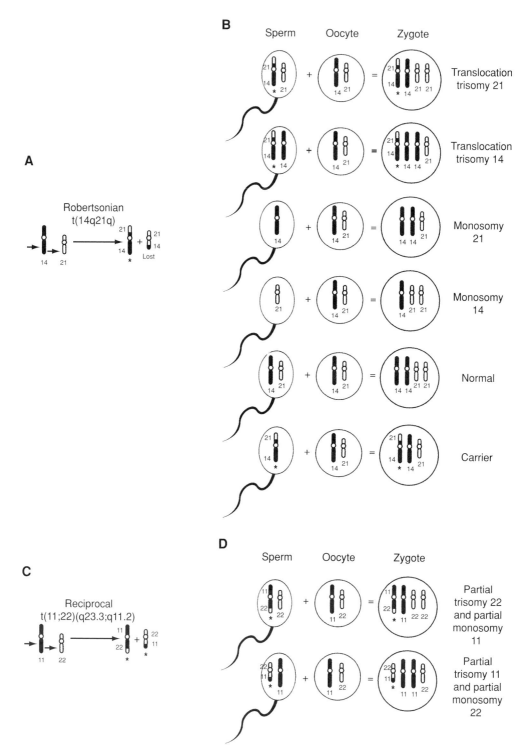

● **Figure 11-2 Translocations. A: Robertsonian t(14q21q).** This is one of the most common Robertsonian translocations found in humans. **B:** The six conditions that may result depending on how chromosomes 14 and 21 segregate
during meiosis when the carrier of the Robertsonian translocation is the male. (*, Robertsonian translocation chromosome.) **C: Reciprocal translocation t(11;22)(q23.3;q11.2).** This is one of the most common reciprocal translocations
found in humans. **D:** The two conditions that may result depending on how chromosomes 11 and 22 segregate during
meiosis when the carrier of the reciprocal translocation is the male. (*, reciprocal translocation chromosome.)

D. **Cytogenetic testing in cancer,** especially the hematopoietic malignancies, is valuable for the diagnosis, prognosis, and management of the disease. Many types of cytogenetic abnormalities are associated with the various types of cancer, but the role of cytogenetic abnormalities in some cancers has been well established. Characterizing the cytogenetic abnormalities can assist with diagnosis, prognosis, and individualization of therapies.

    1. **Acute promyelocytic leukemia (APL) t(15;17)(q22;q21).**

        a. APL t(15;17)(q22;q21) is caused by a reciprocal translocation between chromosomes 15 and 17 with breakpoints at bands q22 and q21, respectively.

        b. This results in a fusion of the **promyelocyte gene (***PML* **gene)** on 15q22 with the **retinoic acid receptor gene (***RARα* **gene)** on 17q21, thereby forming the *pml/rarα* oncogene.

        c. The **PML/RARα oncoprotein** (a transcription factor) blocks the differentiation of promyelocytes to mature granulocytes such that there is continued proliferation of promyelocytes.

        d. **Clinical features include**: coagulopathy and severe bleeding. A rapid cytogenetic diagnosis of this leukemia is essential for patient management, because these patients are at an extremely high risk for stroke.

    2. **Chronic myeloid leukemia (CML) t(9;22)(q34;q11.2)**

        a. CML t(9;22)(q34;q11.2) is caused by a reciprocal translocation between chromosomes 9 and 22 with breakpoints at q34 and q11.2, respectively. The resulting der(22) is referred to as the *Philadelphia chromosome.*

        b. This results in a fusion of the *ABL* **gene** on 9q34 with the *BCR* **gene** on 22q11.1, thereby forming the *abl/bcr* oncogene.

        c. The **ABL/BCR oncoprotein** (a tyrosine kinase) has enhanced tyrosine kinase activity that transforms hematopoietic precursor cells.

        d. **Clinical features include**: increased number of granulocytes in all stages of maturation and many mature neutrophils.

E. **Isochromosomes** occur when the centromere divides transversely (instead of longitudinally) such that one of the chromosome arms is duplicated and the other arm is lost.

    1. **Isochromosome Xq** is a clinical example caused by an isochromosome. **Isochromosome Xq** is caused by a duplication of the q arm and loss of the p arm of chromosome X. Isochromosome Xq is found in 20% of females with **Turner syndrome,** usually as a mosaic cell line along with a 45,X cell line.

    2. **Isochromosome 12p mosaic (Pallister-Killian syndrome).** The occurrence of isochromosomes within any of the autosomes is generally a lethal situation, although isochromosomes for small segments do allow for survival to term. **Clinical features include**: mental retardation, loss of muscle tone, streaks of skin with hypopigmentation, high forehead, coarse facial features, wide space between the eyes, broad nasal bridge, highly arched palate, fold of skin over the inner corner of the eyes, large ears, joint contractures, and cognitive delays.

F. **Chromosome breakage** is caused by breaks in chromosomes due to sunlight (or ultraviolet) irradiation, ionizing irradiation, DNA cross-linking agents, or DNA damaging agents. These insults may cause **depurination of DNA, deamination of cytosine to uracil,** or **pyrimidine dimerization** that must be repaired by DNA repair enzymes.

1. **Xeroderma pigmentosum (XP).**
   a. XP is an autosomal recessive genetic disorder in which the affected individuals are hypersensitive to **sunlight (ultraviolet radiation)**.
   b. XP is caused by the inability to remove pyrimidine dimers due to a genetic defect in one or more of the **nucleotide excision repair enzymes**.
   c. The seven genes involved in the cause of XP are the *XPA*, *ERCC3*, *XPC*, *ERCC2*, *DDB2*, *ERCC4*, and *ERCC5*.
   d. **Clinical features include**: acute sun sensitivity with sunburnlike reaction, severe skin lesions around the eyes and eyelids, and malignant skin cancers (basal and squamous cell carcinomas and melanomas) whereby most individuals die by 30 years of age.

2. **Ataxia-telangiectasia (AT)**
   a. AT is an autosomal recessive genetic disorder involving a gene locus on chromosome 11q22-q23 in which the affected individuals are hypersensitive to **ionizing radiation**.
   b. AT is caused by genetic defects in **DNA recombination repair enzymes**.
   c. The *ATM* gene (AT mutated) is involved in the cause of AT. The *ATM* gene located on chromosome 11q22 encodes for a protein where one region resembles a **PI-3 kinase** (phosphatidylinositol-3 kinase) and another region resembles a **DNA repair enzyme/cell cycle checkpoint protein**.
   d. **Clinical features include**: cerebellar ataxia with depletion of Purkinje cells; progressive nystagmus; slurred speech; oculocutaneous telangiectasia initially in the bulbar conjunctiva followed by the ear, eyelid, cheeks, and neck; immunodeficiency; and death in the second decade of life. A high frequency of structural rearrangements of chromosomes 7 and 14 is the cytogenetic observation with this disease.

Ⅲ Summary Table of Cytogenetic Disorders (Table 11-1)

Ⅳ Selected Photographs of Cytogenetic Disorders (Figure 11-3)

TABLE 11-1	SUMMARY TABLE OF CYTOGENETIC DISORDERS	
Cytogenetic Disorder	**Chromosomal Defect**	**Clinical Features**
Trisomy 21 (Down syndrome)	Aneuploidy; 21 (Down syndrome critical region)	Moderate mental retardation (the leading cause of mental retardation), microcephaly, microphthalmia, colobomata, cataracts and glaucoma, flat nasal bridge, epicanthal folds, protruding tongue, simian crease in hand, increased nuchal skin folds, appearance of an "X" across the face when the baby cries, and congenital heart defects. Alzheimer neurofibrillary tangles and plaques are found in Down syndrome patients over 30 years of age. A condition mimicking acute megakaryocytic leukemia frequently occurs in children with Down syndrome, and they are at increased risk for developing acute lymphoblastic leukemia.

(continued)

TABLE 11-1		**SUMMARY TABLE OF CYTOGENETIC DISORDERS (*Continued*)**
Trisomy 47,XXY (Klinefelter syndrome)	Aneuploidy	Varicose veins, arterial and venous leg ulcer, scant body and pubic hair, male hypogonadism, sterility with fibrosis of seminiferous tubules, marked decrease in testosterone levels, elevated gonadotropin levels, gynecomastia, IQ slightly less than that of siblings, learning disabilities, antisocial behavior, delayed speech as a child, tall stature, and eunuchoid habitus. **Found only in males.**
Monosomy X (Turner syndrome)	Aneuploidy	Short stature, low-set ears, ocular hypertelorism, ptosis, low posterior hairline, webbed neck due to a remnant of a fetal cystic hygroma, congenital hypoplasia of lymphatics causing peripheral edema of hands and feet, shield chest, pinpoint nipples, congenital heart defects, aortic coarctation, female hypogonadism, ovarian fibrous streaks (i.e., infertility), primary amenorrhea, and absence of secondary sex characteristics. **Found only in females.**
Wolf-Hirschhorn syndrome	4p16 deletion	Prominent forehead and broad nasal root ("Greek warrior helmet"), short philtrum, down-turned mouth, congenital heart defects, growth retardation, and severe mental retardation
Cri-du-chat syndrome	5p15 deletion	Round facies, a catlike cry, congenital heart defects, microcephaly, and mental retardation
Prader-Willi syndrome	Paternal 15q11.2-13 microdeletion; imprinting	Poor feeding and hypotonia at birth followed by hyperphagia (insatiable appetite), hypogonadism, obesity, short stature, small hands and feet, behavior problems (rage, violence), and mild to moderate mental retardation
Angelman syndrome	Maternal 15q11.2-13 microdeletion; imprinting	Gait ataxia (stiff, jerky, unsteady, upheld arms), seizures, happy disposition with inappropriate laughter, and severe mental retardation (only 5–10-word vocabulary)
DiGeorge syndrome	22q11.2 microdeletion	Facial anomalies resembling first arch syndrome (micrognathia, low-set ears) due to abnormal neural crest cell migration, cardiovascular anomalies due to abnormal neural crest cell migration during formation of the aorticopulmonary septum, immunodeficiency due to absence of the thymus gland, hypocalcemia due to absence of parathyroid glands
WAGR syndrome	11p14 microdeletion near *WT1* gene	**W**ilms tumor, **a**niridia (absence of the iris), **g**enitourinary abnormalities (e.g., gonadoblastoma), and mental **r**etardation
Robertsonian translocation	t(14q21q) translocation	Translocation trisomy 21 (live birth), translocation trisomy 14 (early miscarriage), monosomy 14 or 21 (early miscarriage), a normal chromosome complement (live birth), or a t(14q21q) carrier (live birth)

(*continued*)

TABLE 11-1		SUMMARY TABLE OF CYTOGENETIC DISORDERS (*Continued*)
Reciprocal translocation	t(11;22)(q23.3;q11.2) translocation	Partial trisomy and partial monosomy
Acute promyelocytic leukemia	t(15;17)(q22;q21) reciprocal transloca- tion forming the *pml/rarα* oncogene	Coagulopathy and severe bleeding. A rapid cytogenetic diagnosis of this leukemia is essential for patient management because these patients are at an extremely high risk for stroke.
Chronic myeloid leukemia	t(9;22)(q34;q11.2) reciprocal transloca- tion forming the *abl/bcr* oncogene (Philadelphia chromosome)	Increased number of granulocytes in all stages of maturation and many mature neutrophils.
Isochromosome Xq	Centromere divides transversely	Found in 20% of females with Turner syndrome
Pallister-Killian syndrome	Centromere divides transversely; isochromosome 12p	Mental retardation, loss of muscle tone, streaks of skin with hypopigmentation, high forehead, coarse facial features, wide space between the eyes, broad nasal bridge, highly arched palate, fold of skin over the inner corner of the eyes, large ears, joint contractures, and cognitive delays
Xeroderma pigmentosa	Chromosome breakage; ultraviolet radiation; affects nucleotide excision repair enzymes	Acute sun sensitivity with sunburnlike reaction, severe skin lesions around the eyes and eyelids, and malignant skin cancers (basal and squamous cell carcinomas and melanomas) whereby most indi- viduals die by 30 years of age
Ataxia- telangiectasia	11q22-q23 chromosome break- age involving the *ATM* gene; ionizing radiation; DNA recombination repair enzymes	Cerebellar ataxia with depletion of Purkinje cells; pro- gressive nystagmus; slurred speech; oculocutaneous telangiectasia initially in the bulbar conjunctiva followed by the ear, eyelid, cheeks, and neck; immunodeficiency; and death in the second decade of life. A high frequency of structural rearrangements of chromosomes 7 and 14 is the cytogenetic observation with this disease.

● **Figure 11-3. Cytogenetic disorders. A: Trisomy 21 (Down syndrome).** Young boy with Down syndrome. Note the flat nasal bridge, prominent epicanthic folds, oblique palpebral fissures, low-set and shell-like ears, and protruding tongue. Other associated features include generalized hypotonia, transverse palmar creases (simian lines), shortening and incurving of the fifth fingers (clinodactyly), Brushfield spots, and mental retardation. **B: Klinefelter syndrome (47,XXY).** Young man with Klinefelter syndrome. Note the hypogonadism, eunuchoid habitus, and gynecomastia. **C: Turner syndrome (45,X).** Three-year-old girl with Turner syndrome. Note the webbed neck due to delayed maturation of lymphatics, short stature, and broad shield chest. **D: Chromosome 4p deletion (Wolf-Hirschhorn syndrome).** Five-year-old boy with Wolf-Hirschhorn syndrome. Note the prominent forehead and broad nasal root ("Greek warrior helmet"), short philtrum, down-turned mouth, and severe mental retardation (IQ = 20). **E: Prader-Willi syndrome.** Ten-year-old boy with PW. Note the hypogonadism, hypotonia, obesity, short stature, and small hands. **F: Angelman syndrome (happy puppet syndrome).** Teenage girl with AS. Note the happy disposition with inappropriate laughter and severe mental retardation (only 5–10-word vocabulary). **G: Acute promyelocytic leukemia t(15;17)(q21;q21).** APL showing abnormal promyelocytes with their characteristic pattern of heavy granulation and bundle of Auer rods. **H: Chronic myeloid leukemia t(9;22)(q34;q11).** CML showing marker granulocytic hyperplasia with neutrophilic precursors at all stages of maturation. Erythroid (red blood cell) precursors are significantly decreased, with none shown in this field. **I: Xeroderma pigmentosa.** Young child with XP. Note the severe facial damage due to exposure to sunlight. **J: Ataxia-telangiectasia.** Eye of a 22-year-old AT patient. Note the striking telangiectasia (permanent dilation of small blood vessels) of the bulbar conjunctiva.

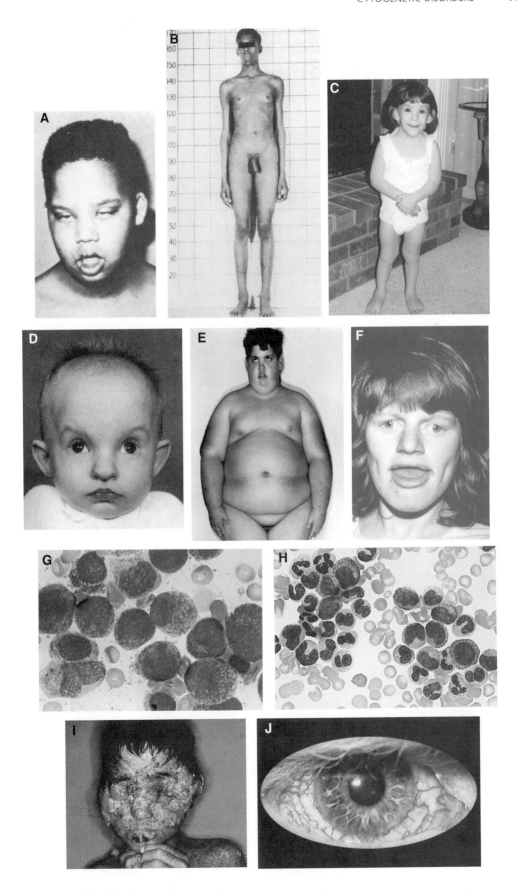

Chapter 12

Population Genetics

I **General Features.** Population genetics is the study of the distributions of genes in populations. In addition, population genetics concerns itself with the factors that maintain or change the frequency of genes (i.e., **gene [allele] frequency**) and frequency of genotypes (i.e., **genotype frequency**) from generation to generation.

A. The **disease frequency** is the frequency that a genetic disease is observed in a population. It is calculated by data-mining hospital records and is expressed as, for example, 1 in 150,000 people.

B. A **gene** is the basic unit of hereditary composed of a finite number of nucleotides arranged in a specific sequence that interacts with the environment to produce a trait.

C. An **allele** is an alternative (or mutated) version of a gene or DNA segment.

D. A **locus** is the physical location of a gene or DNA segment on a chromosome. Since chromosomes are paired in humans, humans have two alleles at each locus.

E. A **polymorphism** is the occurrence of two or more alleles at a specific locus in frequencies greater than can be explained by mutations alone (a polymorphism does not cause a genetic disease).

F. **Single nucleotide polymorphisms** are silent mutations that accumulate in the genome.

G. A **variable number tandem repeat (VNTR) polymorphism** is a polymorphism whereby the number of copies of a tandem repeat sequence of noncoding DNA varies in satellite DNA, minisatellite DNA, or microsatellite DNA.

H. A **genotype** is the gene constitution at a specific locus or the specific mutations present in a given disease.

I. A **phenotype** is the observed physical or clinical findings in a normal person or a disease patient, respectively.

II The Hardy-Weinberg Law

A. HARDY-WEINBERG PRINCIPLES.
1. The Hardy-Weinberg law explains that the allele frequencies do not change from generation to generation in a large population with random mating.

2. The Hardy-Weinberg law explains that the genotype frequency is determined by the relative allele frequencies at that locus.
3. The Hardy-Weinberg law relates the genotype frequency at a locus to the phenotype frequency in a population.

B. HARDY-WEINBERG EQUATION. In a population at equilibrium, for a locus with two alleles (A and a) with allele frequencies of p and q, respectively, the genotype frequencies are determined by the binomial expansion $(p + q = 1)^2$ or $p^2 + 2pq + q^2 = 1$. Therefore, the genotype frequencies are $AA = p^2$, $Aa = 2pq$, and $q^2 = aa$. This is illustrated by the following Punnet square:

	Male Population	
	A (p)	a (q)
Female Population		
A (p)	AA (p^2)	Aa (pq)
a (q)	Aa (pq)	aa (q^2)

C. HARDY-WEINBERG ASSUMPTIONS. The Hardy-Weinberg law applies if the following assumptions are met:
1. **There is a large population so that there is no influence of genetic drift or the founder effect.**
   a. Genetic drift is a fluctuation in allele frequency **due to chance** operating on a small gene pool contained within a small population. In a small population, random factors such as fertility or survival of mutation carriers can cause the allele frequency to rise for reasons other than the mutation itself.
   b. The founder effect is genetic drift that occurs when one of the founders of a new population carries a rare allele that will have a far higher frequency that it did in the larger population from which the new population is derived. Examples include **Huntington disease** in Lake Maracaibo, Venezuela, and **variegate porphyria** in Afrikaner populations of South Africa.
2. **There is random mating (panmixia) with no stratification, assortative mating, or consanguinity.**
   a. Stratification refers to a population where there are subgroups that have remained, for the most part, genetically distinct. An example would be cystic fibrosis, where the carrier frequency of the disorder is 1 in 25 in whites, 1 in 30 in Ashkenazi Jews, 1 in 46 in Hispanics, 1 in 65 in blacks, and 1 in 90 in Asian Americans.
   b. Assortative mating is where the choice of a mate is because of some particular trait. An example of this would be a deaf person preferring another deaf person as a mate.
   c. Consanguinity is where the two mates are related. Progeny from a mating between first cousins is an example where this would apply.
3. **There is a constant mutation rate where genetically lethal alleles (causing death or sterilization) are replaced by new mutations.** If lethal alleles were not replaced by new mutations, the allele frequency would change with each generation and quickly reach zero.

4. **There is no selection for any of the genotypes at a locus.** Selection acts on the fitness of a genotype, with **fitness** (*f*) being a measure of the offspring possessing the genotype that survive to reproduce. A coefficient of selection can be determined, which is 1-*f*.
   a. If the allele determining the genotype is as likely to be present in the next generation as any other allele, then *f* = 1.
   b. If the allele is a genetic lethal, causing death or sterility, then *f* = 0.
   c. If an allele is deleterious so that fewer than normal offspring with the allele are represented in the next generation, then *f* < 1.
5. **There is no migration, no gene flow into or out of the population.** Genes from a migrant population are gradually merged into the gene pool of the population into which they migrated, which can change gene frequencies. Gene flow between populations can slowly change frequencies in both populations, making them more similar to each other. For example, the frequency of sickle cell trait is lower in blacks than in West African populations because of the admixture with other ethnic groups in the United States.

Hardy-Weinberg and Autosomal Dominant Inheritance. In autosomal dominant diseases, homozygosity is exceedingly rare in the population, because this is a lethal genotype most of the time. A good example of this is **achondroplastic dwarfism**. Homozygosity for achondroplastic dwarfism is lethal, so no individuals with this genotype survive to birth. Therefore, individuals in the population with achondroplastic dwarfism are heterozygotes. An exception to this is **Huntington disease**, where homozygosity for the disease has the same clinical severity as the heterozygosity.

Example: Achondroplastic Dwarfism

Question: A recent study of achondroplastic dwarfism documented 7 new cases out of 250,000 in the U.S. population. What is the allele frequency of the achondroplastic dwarfism disease gene in the U.S. population?

Solution: Seven new cases out of 250,000 means that achondroplastic dwarfism occurs in the U.S. population at a disease frequency of 1 in 35,714 or 0.000028 (7/250,000).

All of the genotypes containing the achondroplasia disease gene include only the heterozygotes (Aa;2pq), since homozygosity is lethal. Thus, the frequency of heterozygotes (2pq) is equal to the disease frequency (**2pq = 0.000028**). The allele frequency (p) of the disease gene (A) is usually very small in autosomal dominant diseases, and the allele frequency (q) of the other allele (a) is $\approx$1. Consequently, 2p(1) or 2p equals the disease frequency. This means that 2p(1) = 0.000028 or 2p = 0.000028 or p = 0.000014. In conclusion, the allele frequency (p) of the achondroplasia disease gene is **0.000014 or 1 in 71,428**.

Example: Huntington Disease

Question: Data-mining of the clinical records of a large number of U.S. hospitals indicates that Huntington disease occurs in the U.S. population at a disease frequency of 1 in 10,000 or 0.0001. What is the allele frequency of the Huntington disease gene in the U.S. population?

Solution: All of the genotypes containing the Huntington disease gene include the homozygotes (AA;p^2) and heterozygotes (Aa;2pq). Thus, the frequency of the homozygotes (AA;p^2) and heterozygotes (Aa;2pq) is equal to the disease frequency ($p^2 + 2pq = 0.0001$). The frequency of homozygotes (p^2) is very small (≈ 0), and the allele frequency (q) is ≈ 1. Consequently, 2p(1) or 2p equals the disease frequency. This means that **2p(1) = 0.0001 or 2p = 0.0001 or p = 0.00005**. In conclusion, the allele frequency (p) of the Huntington disease gene is **0.00005 or 1 in 20,000**.

Hardy-Weinberg and Autosomal Recessive Inheritance

A. In autosomal recessive diseases, homozygosity (aa) produces the disease. A good example of this is **sickle cell anemia**. Homozygosity (aa) for sickle cell anemia produces the disease in individuals. Therefore, individuals in the population with sickle cell anemia are homozygotes (aa), and the heterozygotes (Aa) are normal but carriers.

Example: Sickle Cell Anemia

Question: A recent study of sickle cell anemia documented 10 new cases out of 6,250 in the black population. What is the allele frequency (q) of the sickle cell disease gene in the black population? What is the allele frequency (p) of the sickle cell normal gene in the black population? What is the frequency of heterozygote carriers in the black population?

Solution: Ten new cases out of 6,250 means that sickle cell anemia occurs in the black population at a disease frequency of 1 in 625 or 0.0016 (10/6,250). All of the genotypes containing the sickle cell disease gene include the homozygotes (aa;q^2) and heterozygotes (Aa;2pq). The only genotype that produces sickle cell anemia is the homozygous (aa), so $q^2 = 0.0016$. Taking the square root gives **q = 0.04**. In conclusion, the allele frequency (q) of the sickle cell disease gene is **0.04 or 1 in 25**. The allele frequency (p) of the sickle cell normal gene is 1 - q. This means that **p = 1.00 – 0.04 = 0.96**. In conclusion, the allele frequency (p) of the sickle cell normal gene is **0.96 or 1 in 1.04**. The frequency of heterozygote carriers is **2pq**. This means that **2pq = 2(0.96)(0.04) = 0.0768**. In conclusion, the frequency of heterozygote carriers is **0.0768 or 1 in 13**.

B. In rare autosomal recessive diseases, the allele frequency (q) is very small while allele frequency (p) is ≈ 1. In these circumstances, the frequency of heterozygous carriers is approximately equal to 2p.

Example: Congenital Deafness

Question: A recent study of congenital deafness caused by a connexin 26 mutation documented 1 case out of 4,356 in the U.S. population. What is the allele frequency (q) of the connexin 26 mutation in the U.S. population? What is the allele frequency (p) of the connexin 26 normal gene in the U.S. population? What is the frequency of heterozygote carriers in the U.S. population?

Solution: One case out 4,356 means that congenital deafness caused by the connexin 26 mutation occurs in the U.S. population at a frequency of 0.00023 (1/4,356). All of the genotypes containing the connexin 26 mutation include the homozygotes (aa;q^2) and heterozygotes (Aa;2pq). The only genotype that produces congenital deafness is the homozygous (aa), so $q^2 = 0.00023$. Taking the square root gives $q = 0.0151$. In conclusion, the allele frequency (q) of the connexin 26 mutation is **0.0151** or **1 in 66**. The allele frequency (p) of the connexin 26 normal gene is **1 – q**. This means that $p = 1 - 0.0151 = 0.9848$ (or ≈ 1). In conclusion, the allele frequency (p) of the connexin 26 normal gene is **0.9849** or **1 in 1.02**. The frequency of heterozygote carriers is **2pq**. This means that $2pq = 2(1)(0.0151) = 0.0302$. In conclusion, the frequency of heterozygote carries for the connexin 26 mutation is **0.0302** or **1 in 33**.

C. Since only a small proportion of recessive alleles are present in homozygotes, selection does not have much effect on allele frequencies. Even if $f = 0$, it would take many generations to reduce a mutant allele frequency appreciably. In some cases, the heterozygotes have a selective advantage. For example, heterozygous carriers of sickle cell trait have resistance to malaria. Sickle cell trait has its highest carrier frequency in West Africa, where malaria is prevalent.

V Hardy-Weinberg and X-Linked Recessive. In X-linked recessive diseases, males who receive the mutant gene on the X chromosome have the disease. The genotype of a normal male is "$X^A y$" and the genotype of a diseased male is "$X^a y$". A good example of this is **Hunter syndrome (mucopolysaccharidosis II)**.

Example: Hunter Syndrome

Question: A recent study of Hunter syndrome documented 10 new cases out of 1,000,000 over the last 5 years in the U.S. population. What is the allele frequency (q) of the Hunter syndrome disease gene in the U.S. population? What is the allele frequency (p) of the Hunter syndrome normal gene in the U.S. population? What is the frequency of female heterozygote carriers?

Solution: Ten new cases out of 1,000,000 means that Hunter syndrome occurs in the U.S. population at a disease frequency of 1 in 100,000 or 0.00001 (1/100,000). In X-linked recessive diseases, the allele frequency (q) of the Hunter syndrome disease gene equals the disease frequency. This means that **q = 0.00001**. In conclusion, the allele frequency (q) of the Hunter syndrome disease gene is **0.00001 or 1 in 100,000**. The allele frequency (p) of the Hunter syndrome normal gene is **1-q**. This means that **p = 1.00 − 0.00001 = 0.99999** (or ≈1). In conclusion, the allele frequency (p) of the Hunter syndrome normal gene is **0.99999 or 1 in 1.00001**. The frequency of female heterozygote carriers is **2pq**, where p = ≈1. This means that **2pq = 2(1)(0.00001) = 0.00002**. In conclusion, the frequency of female heterozygote carriers is **0.00002 or 1 in 50,000 females**.

VI Summary Table of Hardy-Weinberg Calculations (Table 12-1)

TABLE 12-1	SUMMARY TABLE OF HARDY-WEINBERG CALCULATIONS
	Hardy-Weinberg Calculations Important Equations: $p^2 + 2pq + q^2 = 1$ $p + q = 1$
Autosomal Dominant Inheritance (if homozygote dominants are NOT lethal)	Allele frequency (p) of disease gene (A) $= \dfrac{\text{disease frequency}}{2}$ Allele frequency (q) of normal gene (a) = 1-p
Autosomal Recessive Inheritance	Allele frequency (q) of disease gene (a) = √disease frequency Allele frequency (p) of normal gene (A) = 1-q Frequency of heterozygote carriers = 2pq
X-linked Recessive Inheritance	Allele frequency (q) of disease gene (a) = disease frequency Allele frequency (p) of normal gene (A) = 1-q Frequency of heterozygote carriers = 2pq

Chapter 13

Developmental Genetics

I Causes of Human Birth Defects (Table 13-1)

TABLE 13-1	CAUSES OF HUMAN BIRTH DEFECTS
Causes	**Percentage**
Unknown factors	45
Multifactorial inheritance (environmental and genetic causes combined)	25
Chromosome abnormalities (numerical or structural)	10
Mendelian single gene inheritance	5
Teratogen exposure	5
Uterine factors (e.g., oligohydramnios, uterine fibroids)	3
Twinning	1

II Types of Human Birth Defects

A. MALFORMATION (Genetic-Based). A morphologic defect caused by an **intrinsically abnormal developmental process**. Intrinsic implies that the developmental potential of the primordium is abnormal from the beginning (e.g., a chromosome abnormality of a gamete at fertilization). A malformation occurs during the embryonic period (weeks 3–8 of gestation), when all major organ systems begin to develop (i.e., organogenesis). Malformation may also be due to nutritional deficiencies (e.g., lack of folate in neural tube defects). Malformation examples include polydactyly, oligodactyly, spina bifida, cleft palate, and most kinds of congenital heart malformations.

B. DYSPLASIA (Genetic-Based). A morphologic defect caused by an **abnormal organization of cells into tissues**. A dysplasia occurs during the embryonic period (weeks 3–8 of gestation), when all major organ systems begin to develop (i.e., organogenesis). Dysplasia examples include thanatophoric dwarfism and congenital ectodermal dysplasia.

C. DISRUPTION (Not Genetic-Based). A morphologic defect caused by the breakdown of or interference with an intrinsically normal developmental process. A disruption occurs at any time during gestation. Disruption examples include bowel atresia due to a vascular accidents, amniotic band disruptions, and most cases of porencephaly (cystic lesions of the brain).

D. DEFORMATION (Not Genetic-Based). An abnormality of form or position of a body part caused by mechanical forces that interfere with normal growth or position of the fetus in utero. A deformation occurs usually in the second and third trimester of the pregnancy. Deformation examples include abnormal position of the feet, clubfoot, and abnormal moulding of the head.

Ⅲ **Patterns of Human Birth Defects.** When a patient presents with multiple birth defects, the following patterns may be presented.

A. **SEQUENCE.** A pattern of multiple defects derived from a single known or presumed structural defect or mechanical factor. Sequence examples include Robin sequence and oligohydramnios sequence.

B. **SYNDROME.** A pattern of multiple defects, all of which are pathogenetically related. In clinical genetics, *syndrome* implies a similar cause in all affected individuals. Syndrome examples include Down syndrome, fetal alcohol syndrome, and Marfan syndrome.

C. **POLYTOPIC FIELD DEFECT.** A pattern of multiple defects derived from the disturbance of a single developmental field. Developmental fields are regions of the embryo that develop in a related fashion, although the derivative structures may not be close spatially in the infant or adult. Polytopic field defect examples include holoprosencephaly.

D. **ASSOCIATION.** A pattern of multiple defects that occur more often than expected by chance alone (i.e., nonrandom) but have not yet been classified as a sequence, syndrome, or polytopic field defect. As development genetics advances, many associations will very likely be reclassified as a sequence, syndrome, or polytopic defect. Association examples include abnormal ears associated with renal defects; single umbilical artery associated with heart defects; and the association of vertebral, heart, and kidney defects.

Ⅳ **Determination of the Left/Right (L/R) Axis.** L/R axis determination is established early in embryologic development and is caused by a cascade of paracrine signaling proteins.

A. L/R axis determination begins with the asymmetric (future left-side) expression of the signaling protein **sonic hedgehog (Shh) protein** from the notochord that is located in the midline.

B. This results in the expression of the signaling protein **nodal protein** (a member of the transforming growth factor [TGF]-β family) only on the left side of the embryo (left side, nodal positive; right side, nodal negative) and may be the earliest event in L/R axis determination.

C. After the L/R axis is determined in the embryo, the L/R asymmetry of a number of anatomical organs (e.g., heart, liver, stomach) can then be patterned under the influence of the transcription factor **zinc-finger protein of the cerebellum (ZIC3).**

D. Clinical considerations include the following:
   1. **Situs inversus** describes a right-to-left reversal of viscera. Situs inversus is the mirror image of situs solitus.
   2. **Situs ambiguous (heterotaxy)** describes an uncertain position of viscera.
   3. **Situs solitus** describes normally positioned viscera.
   4. **Cardiac malposition** describes an abnormal position of the heart as a whole and is usually associated with situs inversus or situs ambiguous.
   5. **Dextrocardia with situs solitus (isolated dextrocardia)** is an abnormally positioned heart on the right side of the thorax with the apex pointing to the right and normally positioned viscera. It is usually associated with other severe cardiac abnormalities.
   6. **Dextrocardia with situs inversus or situs ambiguous** is an abnormally positioned heart on the right side of the thorax with the apex pointing to the right and either

a reversal of viscera (situs inversus) or an uncertain position of viscera (situs ambiguous). It is **NOT** usually associated with other severe cardiac abnormalities.

7. **Mesocardia** is an abnormally positioned heart in the midline of the thorax.

8. **Levocardia** is a normally positioned heart on the left side of the thorax with the apex pointing to the left and either a reversal of viscera (situs inversus) or an uncertain position of viscera (situs ambiguous). *Levocardia* is a term used only in conjunction with situs inversus or situs ambiguous.

9. **Conjoined twins.** The incidence of situs inversus in conjoined twins is high. When duplicated structures are joined during a critical period of development, one structure is the mirror image of the other (Bateson's rule).

10. **Primary ciliary dyskinesia (PCD; or immotile cilia syndrome).**

  a. PCD is an autosomal recessive disease involving many mutations in genes that code for various ciliary proteins (e.g., tubulin, dynein). In particular, a number of mutations have been identified in the *DNAH5* gene on chromosome 5p15, which encodes for **dynein axonemal heavy chain 5**, all of which are associated with PCD.

  b. The cilia may be immotile (ciliary immotility), beat abnormally (ciliary dyskinesia), or absent (ciliary aplasia).

  c. **Clinical features of PCD include**: chronic cough, chronic rhinitis, chronic sinusitis, and recurrent sinus/pulmonary infections due to a defect of cilia in the respiratory pathways as well as sterility in males (retarded sperm movement). Situs inversus may occur in individuals with PCD, whereby the individual is said to have **Kartagener syndrome**.

Ⓥ Determination of the Anterior/Posterior (A/P) Axis (Figure 13-1, Table 13-1).

A/P axis determination is established by the formation of the **primitive streak**, which involves the expression of the signaling protein **nodal protein** (a member of the TGF-β family).

A. A large number of gene regulatory proteins called *homeodomain proteins* play a role in determining the normal A/P location of a number of anatomical structures. The genes involved in homeotic mutations are called *homeotic genes*, which are collectively referred to as the *HOM-complex*.

B. All homeotic genes encode for homeodomain proteins, which are gene regulatory proteins. Homeotic genes contain a 180 base pair sequence (called a *homeobox*) that encodes a 60 amino acid–long region (called a *homeodomain*) that binds specifically to DNA segments.

C. A **homeotic mutation** is one in which one body part is substituted for another. Homeotic mutations were first studied in *Drosophila* (e.g., legs sprout from the head in place of antennae).

D. **CLUSTERED HUMAN HOMEOTIC GENES.** There are 39 clustered homeotic genes identified in humans thus far. They are organized into four gene clusters (**HoxA, HoxB, HoxC, and HoxD**) that collectively are called the *Hox-complex*. The Hox-complex is involved in A/P body pattern formation in humans, specifically in the formation of the neural tube, vertebrae, gut tube, genitourinary tract (mesonephric and paramesonephric ducts), limbs, heart tube, and the craniofacial area (inner ear and pharyngeal arch #2).

E. **NONCLUSTERED (Divergent; Dispersed) HUMAN HOMEOTIC GENES.** There are numerous nonclustered homeotic genes that are dispersed randomly throughout the human genome. Nonclustered homeotic genes are involved in the A/P patterning of the mesencephalon and prosencephalon derivatives of the human brain since the clustered Hox-complex genes are never expressed anterior to the rhombencephalon.

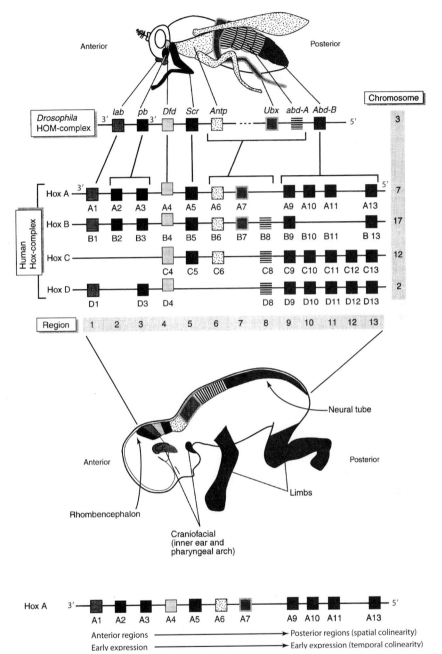

● **Figure 13-1 Schematic diagram demonstrating the relationship between the *Drosophila* HOM-complex and the human Hox-complex.** Each homeotic gene on a chromosome is represented by a shaded box. The expression of the various homeotic genes within body segments of the Drosophila and human fetus are shown by similar shading. The Hox-complex demonstrates two curiosities: (a) the order of Hox genes on each chromosome in a 3′→5′ direction corresponds to the order that the Hox genes are expressed along the A/P axis of the human fetus (called ***spatial colinearity***), that is, Hox genes near the 3′ end are expressed in the anterior region of the embryo whereas Hox genes near the 5′ end are expressed in the posterior region of the embryo; (b) the time of expression of Hox genes on each chromosome occurs in a 3′→5′ direction (called ***temporal colinearity***), that is, Hox genes near the 3′ end are expressed early in embryologic development, and Hox genes near the 5′ end are expressed later in embryologic development. In the human fetus, HoxA-2 is the homeotic gene that is expressed most anterior (up to the rhombencephalon). Please note that **no Hox-complex gene is expressed anterior to the rhombencephalon.** *Exception to the rule:* When looking closely at the sequence of the Hox-A cluster on chromosome 7, HoxA-1 should be the homeotic gene that is expressed most anterior, but it is not. For some reason, the expression of homeotic genes goes out of sequence such that HoxA-2 is expressed most anterior. (lab, labial; pb, proboscipedia; Dfd, deformed; Scr, sex combs reduced; Antp, antennapedia; Ubx, ultrabithorax; abd-A, abdominal-A; Abd-B, abdominal-B.)

Growth and Differentiation (Figure 13-2). The close-range interaction between two or more cells or tissues of different histories is called *induction*. Induction involves an **inducer** (a cell or tissue that produces a signal that changes the behavior of another cell or tissue) and a **responder** (a cell or tissue that is induced). The inducer and responder may interact by either **juxtacrine interactions** or **paracrine interactions**. Juxtacrine interactions occur when cell membrane receptors on the inducer interact with cell membrane receptors on the responder. Paracrine interactions occur when the inducer secretes a protein that diffuses across a small distance and binds to a cell membrane receptor on the responder. These diffusible proteins are called *paracrine factors* or *growth and differentiation factors*. When a paracrine factor binds to a cell membrane receptor on the responder, a series of reactions occur called a *signal transduction pathway*. The end point of a signal transduction pathway is either **activation or deactivation of transcription factors** (i.e., the responder expresses different genes) or the **regulation of the cytoskeleton** (responder changes shape or is permitted to migrate). The paracrine factors are grouped into four major families based on their structure, as indicated below.

A. **FIBROBLAST GROWTH FACTOR (FGF) FAMILY.** The FGF protein family has nine members (**FGF1-FGF9**) along with a number of isoforms. FGFs bind to **FGF receptors (FGFRs)**. The FGFR protein family has four members (**FGFR1-FGFR4**). FGFRs are highly homologous glycoproteins with a signal peptide domain, three immunoglobulin-like domains (IgI-IgIII), a transmembrane domain, and two intracellular tyrosine kinase domains (i.e., **receptor tyrosine kinases**). FGFRs subsequently act through two major signal transduction pathways called the **receptor tyrosine kinase (RTK) pathway** and the **Janus kinase–signal transducers and activators of transcription (JAK/STAT) pathway**.

1. **Achondroplasia (AC).**
   a. AC is an autosomal dominant genetic disorder caused by a missense mutation in the *FGFR3* gene on **chromosome 4p16** whereby a G→A transition occurs at **nucleotide position 1138 (G1138A)**, resulting in a **normal glycine** →**arginine** substitution at position 380 (G380R) in the **transmembrane domain** of FGFR3.
   b. This mutation results in **constitutive activation** of FGFR3 (i.e., a **gain-of-function mutation**), which indicates that FGFR3 normally inhibits bone growth.
   c. However, ≈80% of AC cases are not inherited but result from a **de novo mutation** that occurs during spermatogenesis in the unaffected advanced-aged father. Chances of AC increase with increasing paternal age.
   d. **Skeletal dysplasias** are conditions of abnormal bone growth and typically are called *dwarfisms*. There are **short-limb dysplasias** (short limbs relative to the length of the trunk) and **short-trunk dysplasias** (short trunk relative to the length of the limbs). AC (a short-limb dysplasia) is the most common type of dwarfism (1 in 26,000–40,000 births).
   e. **Clinical features include**: short stature, proximal shortening of arms and legs with redundant skin folds, limitation of elbow extension, trident configuration of hands, bowlegs, thoracolumbar gibbus in infancy, exaggerated lumbar lordosis, large head with frontal bossing, and midface hypoplasia.

2. **Crouzon syndrome (CR).**
   a. CR is an autosomal dominant genetic disorder caused by a missense mutations in the *FGFR2* gene on **chromosome 10q25-q26** that results in either a **normal cysteine**→**tyrosine** substitution at position 342 (C342Y), a **normal cysteine**→**arginine** substitution at position 342 (C342R), a **normal cysteine**→**tryptophan** substitution at position 342 (C342W), or a **normal**

cysteine→phenylalanine substitution at position 278 (C278F) in the **IgIII domain** of FGFR2 (the so-called "cysteine mutational hotspot").
b. These mutations result in **constitutive activation** of FGFR2 (i.e., a **gain-of-function mutation**), which indicates that FGFR2 normally inhibits bone growth.
c. **Clinical features include**: premature craniosynostosis, midface hypoplasia with shallow orbits, ocular proptosis, mandibular prognathism, normal extremities, progressive hydrocephalus, and no mental retardation.

B. THE HEDGEHOG FAMILY. The hedgehog protein family has three members, **sonic hedgehog (Shh), desert hedgehog (Dhh), and indian hedgehog (Ihh)**, which must be complexed to **cholesterol** in order to function. Shh is the most widely used family member. Shh binds to the **patched protein (Ptch)**, which is complexed with the **smoothened protein (Smo)**. Smo subsequently acts through the signal transduction pathway called the *hedgehog pathway*.
1. **Cyclopia.** Some human cyclopia conditions are caused by mutations in genes that encode either Shh or enzymes in the cholesterol biosynthetic pathway. In addition, the teratogens nervine and cyclonamine (both inhibitors of cholesterol biosynthesis) cause cyclopia.
2. **Basal cell nevus syndrome (BCNS).**
   a. BCNS is an autosomal dominant genetic disorder caused by mutation in the *PTCH1* gene for the **patched receptor protein 1** on **chromosome 9q22.3** that binds Shh protein.
   b. In most cases, the mutation is a **loss-of-function mutation** that results in the premature termination of Ptch.
   c. **Clinical features include**: macrocephaly, frontal bossing, hypertelorism, bifid ribs, cleft lip/palate, polydactyly, odontogenic keratocysts in the mandible, palmar and plantar pitting, falx cerebri calcification, and early development of basal cell carcinomas.

C. THE WNT (Wingless and Integrated) FAMILY. The Wnt protein family has 19 members (Wnt1-Wnt19) that must be complexed to a **lipid** in order to function. Wnts bind to the **frizzled receptor (FR)** and to the **lipoprotein-related receptor 5 (LRP-5)**. FR and LRP-5 subsequently act through the signal transduction pathway called the *canonical Wnt pathway*. The Wnts play a role in muscle, gonad, kidney, limb, and bone formation.

D. THE TGF-β SUPERFAMILY. The TGF-β protein superfamily has >30 members, including the **TGF-β family, activin family, bone morphogenetic proteins (BMPs), Vg1 family, glial-derived neurotrophic factor (GDNF)**, and **müllerian inhibitory factor**. These members binds to the **type I TGF-β receptor** and **type II TGF-β receptor (TGF-βR)**. TGF-βR subsequently acts through the signal transduction pathway called the *SMAD pathway*. The TGF-β superfamily members play a role in formation of the extracellular matrix; regulation of mitosis; duct formation in kidney, lungs, and salivary glands; bone formation; apoptosis; cell migration; neural tube polarity; sperm formation; enteric neuron differentiation; and sex determination.

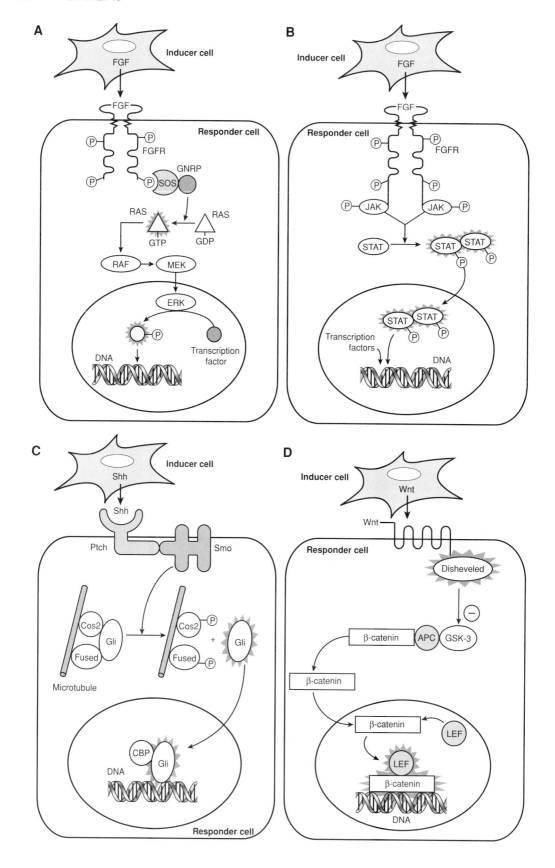

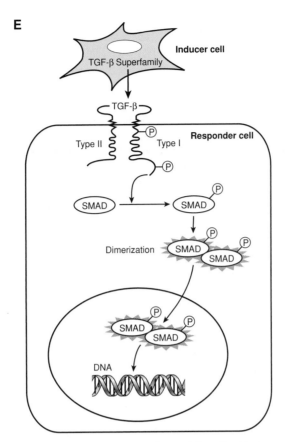

● **Figure 13-2 Signal transduction pathways. A: RTK pathway.** When fibroblast growth factor (*FGF*) binds to the fibroblast growth factor receptor (*FGFR*), autophosphorylation of FGFR occurs. This is recognized by *SOS* adaptor protein, which activates guanine nucleotide releasing factor (*GNRP*). GNRP activates the G protein *RAS* by exchanging a PO_4^{2-} from *GTP* to transform the bound *GDP* to GTP (RAS-GDP→RAS-GTP). RAS-GTP activates the kinase *RAF*, which activates the kinase *MEK*, which then activates the kinase *ERK*. ERK enters the nucleus and phosphorylates transcription factors, which then modulate gene expression activity. **B: JAK/STAT pathway.** When FGF binds to other receptors linked to *JAK*, the receptors dimerize and the JAK proteins phosphorylate each other and the dimerized receptors, which activates the dormant kinase activity of the receptor. The activated receptor phosphorylates *STAT*, which allows STAT to dimerize. The activated dimerized STAT enters the nucleus and along with other transcription factors modulates gene expression activity. **C: Hedgehog pathway.** When sonic hedgehog (*Shh*) protein binds to the patched (*Ptch*) protein that is complexed to the smoothened (*Smo*) protein, *Gli* is released from microtubules probably by the phosphorylation of *Cos 2* and *Fused*. Gli enters the nucleus, binds to *CBP*, and acts as a transcription factor, which then modulates gene expression activity. **D: Wnt pathway.** When *Wnt* protein binds to the frizzled receptor (*FR*), *Disheveled* protein is activated, inhibiting glycogen synthase kinase 3 (*GSK-3*). When GSK-3 is inhibited, β-catenin dissociates from adenomatosis polyposis coli (*APC*) protein. β-catenin enters the nucleus, binds to late expression factor (*LEF*), and acts as a transcription factor, which then modulates gene expression activity. **E: SMAD (Sma protein and Mad protein) pathway.** When a TGF-β superfamily protein binds to the type II TGF-β receptor, the type II TGF-β receptor binds the type I TGF-β receptor and phosphorylates it. The phosphorylated type I and type II TGF-β receptor complex phosphorylates the *SMAD* protein. The phosphorylated SMAD proteins dimerize. The activated dimerized SMAD proteins enter the nucleus and modulate gene expression activity.

VII **Formation of the Extracellular Matrix (ECM) (Figure 13-3A).** The ECM consists of various macromolecules secreted by cells (e.g., mesenchymal cells, fibroblasts, chondroblasts, osteoblasts) and forms a noncellular material in the interstices between cells. The ECM is not inert but instead plays an important embryologic role in cell adhesion, cell migration, and formation of epithelial sheets. The ECM consists of proteoglycans, glycoproteins, and fibers (i.e., collagen and elastic fibers).

A. PROTEOGLYCANS. Proteoglycans bind paracrine factors (e.g., FGF, Shh, Wnt, and TGF-β superfamily) secreted by an inducer cell and deliver the paracrine factors in high concentration to their respective receptors located on the responder cell. Specific proteoglycans include **aggrecan**, **betaglycan**, **decorin**, **perlecan**, and **syndecan-1**.

B. GLYCOPROTEINS (Figure 13-3B,C). Glycoproteins play a role in cell migration and modulation of gene expression activity. Specific glycoproteins include **fibronectin**, **laminin**, **chondronectin**, **osteocalcin**, **osteopontin**, and **bone sialoprotein**.
1. Fibronectin is a 460 kDa glycoprotein dimer with a heparin-binding domain, collagen-binding domain, a fibrin-binding domain, and a RGD sequence domain that binds to cell receptors.
2. Fibronectin binds to the **fibronectin receptor (FBR)**. FBR is unique in that it binds fibronectin extracellularly and the **actin microfilament network** intracellularly, thereby integrating the ECM with the intracellular matrix (these type of receptors are commonly referred to as *integrins*). When fibronectin binds FBR, the actin microfilament network is activated and **cell migration** occurs.
3. FBR is linked to the **RTK pathway** by caveolin and Fyn proteins.

C. COLLAGEN AND ELASTIC FIBERS. Collagen is a family of proteins consisting of three polypeptide **α-chains** that form a triple-stranded helical structure. There are 25 distinct collagen α-chain genes. However, only ≈20 different types of collagens (types I–XX) have been isolated. **Elastic fibers** consist of an amorphous core of the **elastin** protein surrounded by microfibrils of the **fibrillin** protein.

D. Osteogenesis imperfecta (OI).
1. OI (types I–IV) is an autosomal dominant genetic disorder caused by a mutation either in the *COL1A1* gene on **chromosome 17q21.3-q22** for collagen **α-1(I)chain protein** or the *COL1A2* gene on **chromosome 7q22.1** for collagen **α-2(I) chain protein**.
2. Type I OI is most commonly caused by a **frameshift mutation** or a **RNA splicing mutation** (that forms a premature STOP codon, shifts a reading frame, or produces unstable messenger RNAs [mRNAs]).
3. Types II, III, and IV OI are most commonly caused by a **missense mutation**, resulting in a normal glycine→serine, normal glycine→arginine, normal glycine→cysteine, or normal glycine→tryptophan substitution that alters the structure of the α1(I)-chain or the α2(I)-chain since glycine is necessary for normal folding of the collagen helix.
4. OI is a group of disorders (types I–VII) with a continuum ranging from perinatal lethality→severe skeletal deformities→nearly asymptomatic individuals. Nearly 40% of type I OI-affected individuals (i.e., milder forms of OI) inherit a mutant gene from an affected parent, whereas ≈60% have a de novo mutation. Nearly 100% of types II and III OI-affected individuals (i.e., more severe forms of OI) have a de novo mutation.

5. **Clinical features include**: extreme bone fragility with spontaneous fractures, short stature with bone deformities, grey or brown teeth, blue sclera of the eye, and progressive postpubertal hearing loss. Milder forms of OI may be confused with child abuse. Severe forms of OI are fatal in utero or during the early neonatal period.

E. CLASSIC-TYPE EHLERS-DANLOS SYNDROME (EDS).

1. EDS is an autosomal dominant genetic disorder caused by a mutation either in the *COL5A1* **gene** on **chromosome 9q34.2-q34.3** for **collagen α-1(V) chain protein** or the *COL5A2* **gene** on **chromosome 2q31** for **collagen α-2(V) chain protein**.

2. EDS is most commonly caused by a **nonsense mutation, frameshift mutation,** or a **RNA splicing mutation** (that forms a premature STOP codon, shifts a reading frame, or produces unstable mRNAs).

3. Nearly 50% of EDS-affected individuals inherit a mutant gene from an affected parent, whereas ≈50% have a de novo mutation.

4. **Clinical features include**: extremely stretchable and fragile skin, hypermobile joints, aneurysms of blood vessels, rupture of the bowel, and widened atrophic scars.

F. MARFAN SYNDROME (MFS).

1. MFS is an autosomal dominant genetic disorder caused by a mutation in the *FBN1* **gene** on **chromosome 15q21.1** for the **fibrillin-1** protein, which is an essential component of **elastic fibers**.

2. MFS is caused by >200 different mutations, and no common mutation is associated with any population. Nearly 75% of MFS-affected individuals inherit a mutant gene from an affected parent, whereas ≈25% have a de novo mutation.

3. **Clinical features include**: unusually tall individuals, exceptionally long and thin limbs, pectus excavatum ("hollow chest"), ectopia lentis (dislocation of the lens), severe nearsightedness (myopia), and dilatation or dissection of the aorta at the level of the sinuses of Valsalva (which may lead to cardiomyopathy or even a rupture of the aorta, dural ectasia, and mitral valve prolapse).

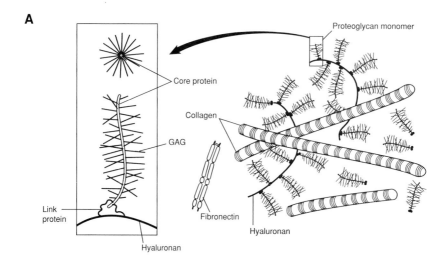

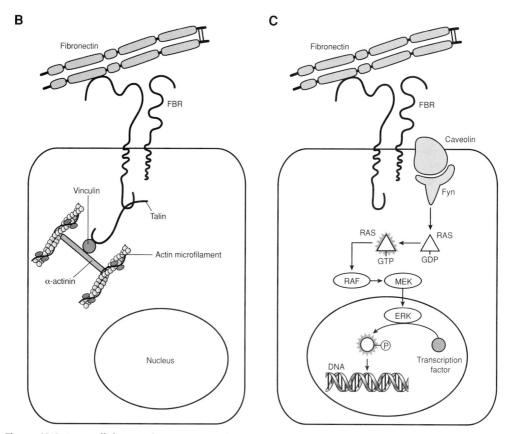

● **Figure 13-3 Extracellular matrix. A:** A proteoglycan monomer and its relationship to hyaluronan. Proteoglycans consist of a core protein, which binds many side chains of glycosaminoglycans (*GAG*), and a link protein, which binds hyaluronic acid. GAGs are highly sulfated (SO_4^{2-}) and consist of repeating disaccharide units of a hexosamine (e.g., N-acetylglucosamine, N-acetylgalactosamine) and a uronic acid (e.g., glucuronic acid). Specific GAGs include hyaluronan, chondroitin sulfate, keratan sulfate, dermatan sulfate, and heparan sulfate. The proteoglycan aggregates interact with various glycoproteins (e.g., fibronectin) and fibers (e.g., collagen). **B:** The pathway by which the extracellular glycoprotein fibronectin binds to the fibronectin receptor (*FBR*) and causes cell migration by activating the actin microfilament network. **C:** The pathway by which the extracellular glycoprotein fibronectin binds to the fibronectin receptor (*FBR*) and causes modulation of gene expression activity via the RTK pathway. (See figure 13-2A for complete pathway).

Neural Crest Cell Migration. The neural crest cells differentiate from cells located along the lateral border of the neural plate that is mediated by **BMP-4** and **BMP-7**. The differentiation of neural crest cells is marked by the expression of *slug* (a zinc-finger transcription factor), which characterizes cells that break away from the neuroepithelium of the neural plate and migrate into the extracellular matrix as mesenchymal cells. Neural crest cells undergo a prolific migration throughout the embryo (both the cranial region and trunk region) and ultimately differentiate into a wide array of adult cells and structures. *Neurocristopathy* is a term used to describe any disease related to maldevelopment of neural crest cells.

A. WAARDENBURG SYNDROME (WS).

1. WS is an autosomal dominant genetic disorder caused by a mutation in either the *PAX3* gene on chromosome 2q35 (for type I WS) for the **paired box protein PAX3** or the *MITF* gene on chromosome 3p14.3-p14.1 (for type II WS). Paired box protein PAX3 is one of a family of nine human *PAX genes* coding for **DNA-binding transcription factors** that are expressed in the early embryo.

2. The mutations of the *PAX3* gene include **missense, nonsense, frameshift, whole gene deletions, intragenic deletions,** and **RNA splicing mutations**, all of which result in a **loss-of-function mutation.**

3. Nearly 90% of PAX3 affected individuals inherit a mutant gene from an affected parent, whereas ≈10% have a de novo mutation.

4. **Clinical features include**: dystopia canthorum (malposition of the eyelid), a growing together of eyebrows, lateral displacement of lacrimal puncta, a broad nasal root, heterochromia of the iris, congenital deafness or hearing impairment, and piebaldism including a white forelock and a triangular area of hypopigmentation.

B. NONSYNDROMIC CONGENITAL INTESTINAL AGANGLIONOSIS (Hirschsprung Disease; HSCR).

1. HSCR is an autosomal dominant genetic disorder associated with mutations in six different genes: *RET* (**re**arranged **d**uring **t**ransfection) gene on chromosome 10q11.2 for a **receptor tyrosine kinase** (≈90% of HSCR cases), *GDNF* gene on chromosome 5p13.1-p14 for **glial cell line–derived neurotrophic factor**, *NRTN* gene on chromosome 19p13.3 for **neurturin**, *EDNRB* gene on chromosome 13q22 for the **endothelin B receptor**, *EDN3* gene on chromosome 20q13.2-q13.3 for **endothelin-3**, and the *ECE1* gene on chromosome 1p36.1 for **endothelin-converting enzyme.**

2. **Clinical features include**: arrest of the caudal migration of neural crest cells resulting in the absence of ganglionic cells in the myenteric and submucosal plexuses, abdominal pain and distention, inability to pass meconium within the first 48 hours of life, gushing of fecal material during a rectal digital exam, constipation, emesis, a loss of peristalsis in the colon segment distal to the normal innervated colon, and failure of the internal anal sphincter to relax following rectal distention (i.e., abnormal rectoanal reflex).

C. OROFACIAL CLEFTING.

1. Orofacial clefting is a multifactorial genetic disorder involving the following genes crucial to midface development:

   a. *DLX 1-6* (**d**istal **l**ess homeobo**x**) gene family on chromosomes 2q32, 2cen-q33, 17q21.3-q22, 17q21.33, 7q22, and 7q22, respectively, for various **homeodomain gene regulatory proteins.**

b. *SHH* gene on chromosome 7q36 for the Shh protein.

c. *TGF-α* gene on chromosome 2p13 for the TGF-α variant protein.

d. *TGF-β* gene on chromosome 14q24 for the TGF-β protein.

e. *IRF-6* (interferon regulatory factor) gene on chromosome 1q32.3-q41 for the IRF6 transcription factor.

2. Orofacial clefting has a **multifactorial inheritance** (i.e., a genetic component involving various genes and an environmental component). Orofacial clefting is a genetically complex event where 2–20 different genes are involved; a single gene mutation causing orofacial clefting probably does not occur.

3. Environmental factors that may play a role in orofacial clefting involve exposure of the fetus to **phenytoin, sodium valproate,** and **methotrexate.**

4. The most common craniofacial birth defect is the orofacial cleft, which consists of **cleft lip with or without cleft palate (CL/P)** or **isolated cleft palate (CP).** CL/P and CP are distinct birth defects based on their embryologic formation, etiology, candidate genes, and recurrence risk.

a. CL/P is more common than CP and varies by ethnicity. CL/P is found at a high level in American Indians and Asians (1/500 births), intermediate level in whites (1/1,000 births), a low level in American blacks (1/2,000 births), and occurs more frequently in males.

b. CP occurs in 1 in 2,500 births, does not show ethnic variation, and occurs more frequently in females.

D. TREACHER COLLINS SYNDROME (TCS; or Mandibulofacial Dysostosis).

1. TCS is an autosomal dominant genetic disorder caused by a mutation in the *TCOFI* **gene** on **chromosome 5q32-q33.1** for the **treacle protein.** The treacle protein is a nucleolar protein related to the nucleolar phosphoprotein **Nopp140,** both of which contain **LIS1 motifs** leading to the speculation of **microtubule dynamics** involvement. In addition, treacle interacts with the small nucleolar ribonucleoprotein **hNop56p** leading to the speculation of **ribosomal biogenesis** involvement.

2. More than 100 mutations in the *TCOF1* gene have been identified, with **frameshift mutations** forming a premature STOP codon being the most common type of mutation.

● **Figure 13-4 Birth defects associated with various developmental processes. A: Dextrocardia with situs solitus (isolated dextrocardia).** Radiograph shows the heart on the right side of the thorax with the cardiac apex pointing to the right. Note that the stomach is on the normal left side, indicated by the gastric bubble (*arrow*). **B: Primary ciliary dyskinesia (immotile cilia syndrome).** Electron micrograph shows a cilium from an individual with PCD where the outer dynein arms are absent and with three abnormal single microtubules (*M*) instead of the normal 9 + 2 arrangement. **C: Achondroplasia.** A boy with short stature, short limbs (particularly in the proximal portions), short fingers, disproportionate trunk, bowed legs, relatively large head, prominent forehead, and deep nasal ridge. **D: Crouzon syndrome. E: Basal cell nevus syndrome.** A man with pigmented facial basal cell carcinomas with postsurgical scars and a glabellar graft. **F: Osteogenesis imperfecta.** Radiograph shows multiple bone fractures of the upper and lower limbs resulting in an accordionlike shortening of the limbs. **G: Ehlers-Danlos syndrome.** The extremely stretchable skin of the infant. **H: Marfan syndrome.** A girl with an unusually tall stature, exceptionally long limbs, and arachnodactyly (elongated hands and feet with very slender digits). **I: Waardenburg syndrome.** A young boy with a white forelock of hair, partial albinism, heterochromia of the iris, and lateral displacement of the medial canthi. **J: Nonsyndromic congenital intestinal aganglionosis (Hirschsprung disease).** Radiograph after barium enema of a patient with Hirschsprung disease. The upper segment of the normal colon (∗) is distended with fecal material. The lower segment of the colon (∗∗) is narrow. The lower segment is the portion of the colon where the ganglionic cells in the myenteric and submucosal plexuses are absent, and peculiar contractions are observed. This case shows a high transition zone (*T*) between the normal colon and aganglionic colon. The *arrows* indicate a long segment of aganglionic descending colon. **K: Unilateral cleft lip and cleft palate. L: Treacher Collins syndrome (mandibulofacial dysostosis).** Underdevelopment of the zygomatic bones, mandibular hypoplasia, lower eyelid colobomas, downward-slanting palpebral fissures, and malformed external ears (note the hearing aid cord).

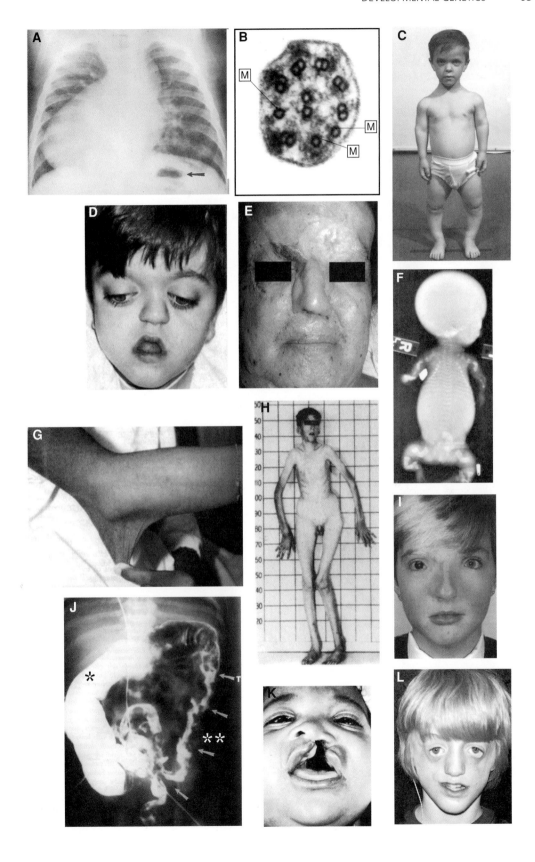

3. Nearly 40% of TCS-affected individuals inherit a mutant gene from an affected parent, whereas ≈60% have a de novo mutation.
4. TCS belongs to a category of **first arch syndromes** that result from a lack of neural crest cell migration into **pharyngeal arch 1** and produce various facial anomalies. There are two well-described first arch syndromes: TCS and **Pierre Robin syndrome**.
5. **Clinical features include**: hypoplasia of the zygomatic bones and mandible resulting in midface hypoplasia, micrognathia, and retrognathia; external ear abnormalities including small, absent, malformed, or rotated ears; and lower eyelid abnormalities including coloboma.

IX   Photographs of Birth Defects Associated with Various Developmental Processes (Figure 13-4)

Chapter 14

Metabolic Genetics

❶ Introduction

A. Metabolic reactions within various biochemical pathways are controlled by **enzymes** that increase the reaction rate by a million fold. In general, metabolic genetic disorders are caused by mutations in genes that encode for enzymes of various biochemical pathways.

B. Most metabolic genetic disorders are **autosomal recessive disorders** whereby individuals with two mutant alleles (homozygous recessive) demonstrate clinically apparent, phenotypic errors in metabolism. A heterozygote is generally normal because the one normal allele produces enough enzymatic activity to maintain normal metabolism.

C. The parents of a proband are obligate heterozygotes whereby each parent carries one mutant allele and is asymptomatic.

D. For example, in the case of galactosemia (GAL), the risk to the siblings of the proband is a 25% chance of having the disorder (gg), a 50% chance of being a normal heterozygote carrier (Gg), and a 25% chance of being a normal homozygous individual (GG).

E. As another example, in the case of GAL, if one parent has the disorder (gg) and the other parent is a normal homozygous individual (GG), then their children are obligate normal heterozygote carriers (Gg). If one parent has GAL (gg) and the other parent is a normal heterozygote individual (Gg), then their children have a 50% chance of having the disorder (gg) and a 50% chance of being a normal heterozygote carrier (Gg).

❷ Metabolic Genetic Disorders Involving Carbohydrate Pathways (Table 14-1)

A. GALACTOSEMIA.
   1. GAL is an autosomal recessive genetic disorder caused by various **missense mutations** in the *GALT* gene on **chromosome 9p13** for **galactose-1-phosphate uridylyltransferase (GALT)**, which catalyzes the reaction galactose-1-phosphate→glucose-1-phosphate.
   2. The various missense mutations result either in a **normal glutamine→arginine** substitution at position 188 (Q188R), prevalent in northern Europe; a **normal serine→leucine** substitution at position 135 (S135L), prevalent in Africa; or a **normal lysine→asparagine** substitution at position 285 (K285N), prevalent in Germany, Austria, and Croatia.
   3. The **Duarte variant allele** is caused by a missense mutation that results in a normal asparagine→aspartate substitution at position 314 (N314D), imparting instability to GALT, whereby affected individuals have ≈5% GALT activity compared with normal individuals.

4. Clinical features include: feeding problems in the newborn, failure to thrive, hypoglycemia, hepatocellular damage, bleeding diathesis, jaundice, and hyperammonemia. Sepsis with *Escherichia coli*, shock, and death may occur if the galactosemia is not treated.

B. ASYMPTOMATIC FRUCTOSURIA (AF; Essential Fructosuria).

1. AF is an autosomal recessive genetic disorder caused by a mutation in the *KHK* gene on chromosome 2p23.3-p23.2 for **ketohexokinase (or fructokinase)**, which catalyzes the reaction fructose→fructose-1-phosphate.
2. **Clinical features include**: presence of fructose in the urine.

C. HEREDITARY FRUCTOSE INTOLERANCE (HFI; Fructosemia).

1. HFI is an autosomal recessive genetic disorder caused by a mutation in the *ALDOB* gene on **chromosome 9q21.3-q22.2** for **fructose 1-phosphate aldolase B**, which catalyzes the reaction fructose 1-phosphate→dihydroxyacetone phosphate + D-glyceraldehyde.
2. The most likely mechanism causing the clinical features of HFI is that the PO_4^{3-} group becomes sequestered on fructose and therefore is not available for ATP synthesis.
3. **Clinical features include**: failure to thrive, fructosuria, hepatomegaly, jaundice, aminoaciduria, metabolic acidosis, lactic acidosis, low urine ketones, recurrent hypoglycemia, and vomiting at the age of weaning when fructose or sucrose (a disaccharide that is hydrolyzed to glucose and fructose) is added to the diet. Infants and adults are asymptomatic until they ingest fructose or sucrose.

D. LACTOSE INTOLERANCE (LI; Lactase Nonpersistence; Adult-type Hypolactasia).

1. LI is an autosomal recessive genetic disorder associated with short tandem repeat polymorphisms (STRPs) in the promoter region that affects transcriptional activity of the *LCT* gene on **chromosome 2q21** for **lactase-phlorizin hydrolase**, which catalyzes the reaction lactose→glucose + galactose.
2. These STRPs in the human population lead to two distinct phenotypes: **lactase-persistent** individuals and **lactase-nonpersistent** individuals.
3. All healthy newborn children up to the age of ≈5–7 years of age have high levels of lactase-phlorizin hydrolase activity, so they can digest large quantities of lactose present in milk.
4. Northern European adults (particularly Scandinavian) retain high levels of lactase-phlorizin activity and are known as **lactase persistent** and therefore **lactose tolerant**.
5. However, a majority of the world's adults (particularly Africa and Asia) lose the high levels of lactase-phlorizin activity and are known as **lactase nonpersistent** and therefore **lactose intolerant**.
6. **Clinical findings of lactose intolerance include**: diarrhea; crampy abdominal pain localized to the periumbilical area or lower quadrant; flatulence; nausea; vomiting; audible borborygmi; stools that are bulky, frothy, and watery; and bloating after milk or lactose consumption.

E. GLYCOGEN STORAGE DISEASE TYPE I (GSDI; von Gierke).

1. GSDIa is an autosomal recessive genetic disorder caused by ≈85 different mutations in the *G6PC* gene on **chromosome 17q21** for **glucose-6-phosphatase**, which catalyzes the reaction glucose-6-phosphate→glucose + phosphate.
2. GSDIb is an autosomal recessive genetic disorder caused by ≈78 different mutations in the *SLC37A4* gene on **chromosome 11q23** for **glucose-6-phosphate**

translocase, which transports glucose-6-phosphate into the lumen of the endoplasmic reticulum.

3. GSDIa is commonly (32% of cases in the white population and 93%–100% of cases in the Jewish population) caused by a **missense mutation** that results in a **normal arginine → cysteine** substitution at position 83 (R83C). GSDIb is commonly (15% of cases in the white population and 30% of cases in the German population) caused by a **missense mutation** that results in a **normal glycine → cysteine** substitution at position 339 (G339C).

4. **Clinical features include:** accumulation of glycogen and fat in the liver and kidney resulting in hepatomegaly and renomegaly, severe hypoglycemia, lactic acidosis, hyperuricemia, hyperlipidemia, hypoglycemic seizures, doll-like faces with fat cheeks, relatively thin extremities, short stature, protuberant abdomen, and neutropenia with recurrent bacterial infections.

F. GLYCOGEN STORAGE DISEASE TYPE V (GSDV; McArdle Disease).

1. GSDV is an autosomal recessive genetic disorder caused by ≈46 different mutations in the *PYGM* gene on **chromosome 11q13** for **muscle glycogen phosphorylase,** which initiates glycogen breakdown by removing α1,4 glucosyl residues from the outer branches of glycogen with liberation of glucose-1-phosphate.

2. GSDV is commonly caused by either a nonsense mutation that results in a **normal arginine → nonsense** at position 49 (R49X) causing a premature STOP codon (90% of cases in U.S. and European populations) or a missense mutation that results in a **normal glycine → serine** substitution at position 204 (G204S; 10% of cases in U.S. and European populations).

3. **Clinical features include:** exercise-induced muscle cramps and pain, "second wind" phenomenon with relief of myalgia and fatigue after a few minutes of rest, episodes of myoglobinuria, increased resting basal serum creatine kinase (CK) activity, and onset typically occurring at around 20–30 years of age; in preadolescents, clumsiness, lethargy, slow movement, and laziness.

G. OTHER GLYCOGEN STORAGE DISEASES. These include: glycogen storage disease type II (GSDII; Pompe), glycogen storage disease type IIIa (GSDIIIa; Cori), glycogen storage disease type IV (GSDIV; Andersen), glycogen storage disease type VI (GSDVI; Hers), and glycogen storage disease type VII (GSDVII; Tarui).

Ⅲ Metabolic Genetic Disorders Involving Amino Acid Pathways (Table 14-2)

A. PHENYLALANINE HYDROXYLASE (PAH) DEFICIENCY.

1. PAH deficiency is an autosomal recessive genetic disorder caused by a mutation in the *PAH* gene on **chromosome 12q23.2** for **phenylalanine hydroxylase,** which catalyzes the reaction phenylalanine → tyrosine.

2. PAH deficiency is caused by missense (most common; 62% of cases), small deletion (13% of cases), RNA splicing (11% of cases), silent (6% of cases), nonsense (5% of cases), or insertion (2% of cases) mutations.

3. PAH deficiency results in an intolerance to the dietary intake of phenylalanine (an essential amino acid). This produces a variability in metabolic phenotypes including **classic phenylketonuria (PKU), non-PKU hyperphenylalaninemia,** and **variant PKU.** This variability in metabolic phenotypes is caused primarily by different mutations in the *PAH* gene that result in variations in the kinetics of phenylalanine uptake, permeability of the blood–brain barrier, and protein folding.

4. Classic PKU is associated with the complete absence of PAH and is the most severe of the three types of PAH deficiency.

5. **Clinical features of classic PKU include**: no physical signs are apparent in neonates with PAH deficiency; diagnosis is based on detection of elevated plasma PAH concentration ($>1,000$ umol/L for classic PKU) and normal BH_4 cofactor metabolism; a dietary phenylalanine tolerance of <500 mg/day; and untreated children with classic PKU show impaired brain development, microcephaly, epilepsy, severe mental retardation, behavioral problems, depression, anxiety, musty body odor, and skin conditions like eczema.

B. HEREDITARY TYROSINEMIA TYPE I (TYRI).

1. **TYRI** is an autosomal recessive genetic disorder caused by a mutation in the *FAH* gene on **chromosome 15q23-q25** for **fumarylacetoacetate hydrolase**, which catalyzes the reaction fumarylacetoacetic acid→fumarate + acetoacetate.

2. **TYRI** is caused by either a missense mutation that results in a **normal proline→leucine** substitution at position 261 (P261L) or RNA splicing mutations IVS12+5 G→A, IVS6-1 G→T, and IVS7-6 T→G. The P261L, IVS12+5 G→A, IVS6-1 G→T, and IVS7-6 T→G mutations account for 60% of cases in the U.S. population. The P261L mutation accounts for 100% of cases in the Ashkenazi Jewish population. The IVS12 + 5 G→A accounts for 88% of cases in the French Canadian population.

3. **Clinical features include**: diagnosis is based on detection of elevated plasma succinylacetone concentration, elevated plasma tyrosine, methionine, and phenylalanine concentrations as well as elevated urinary tyrosine metabolite (e.g., hydroxyphenylpyruvate) concentration and elevated urinary δ-aminolevulinic acid; cabbagelike odor; untreated children with HTI show severe liver dysfunction, renal tubular dysfunction, growth failure, and rickets.

C. MAPLE SYRUP URINE DISEASE (MSUD).

1. MSUD is an autosomal recessive genetic disorder cause by >60 different mutations in either the *BCKDHA* gene on **chromosome 19q13.1-q13.2** for the **E1α subunit of the branched-chain ketoacid dehydrogenase complex (BCKD)**, the *BCKDHB* gene on **chromosome 6q14** for the **E1β subunit of BCKD**, or the *DBT* gene on **chromosome 1p31** for the **E2 subunit of BCKD**, all of which catalyze the second step in the degradation of branched-chain amino acids (e.g., leucine, isoleucine, and valine).

2. The BCKD enzyme is an enzyme complex found in the mitochondria.

3. **Clinical features include**: untreated children with MSUD show maple syrup odor in cerumen 12–24 hours after birth; elevated plasma branched-chain amino acid concentration; ketonuria; irritability; poor feeding by 2–3 days of age; deepening encephalopathy including lethargy, intermittent apnea, opisthotonus, and stereotyped movements like "fencing" and "bicycling" by 4–5 days of age; and acute leucine intoxication (leucinosis) associated with neurologic deterioration due to the ability of leucine to interfere with the transport of other large neutral amino acids across the blood–brain barrier, thereby reducing the amino acid supply to the brain.

Ⅳ Metabolic Genetic Disorders Involving the Urea Cycle Pathway (Table 14-3)

A. The urea cycle produces the amino acid arginine (this is the only source of endogenous arginine) and clears waste nitrogen resulting from the metabolism of proteins and dietary intake (this is the only pathway for waste nitrogen clearance). The waste nitrogen is converted to ammonia (NH_4) and transported to the liver.

B. The severity of these disorders are influenced by the position of the defective enzyme in the urea cycle pathway and the severity of the enzyme defect (partial activity vs. absent activity).

C. Since the urea cycle is the only pathway for waste nitrogen clearance, clinical symptoms develop very rapidly.

D. **Clinical features include**: infants initially appear normal but then rapidly develop hyperammonemia, cerebral edema, lethargy, anorexia, hyperventilation or hypoventilation, hypothermia, seizures, neurologic posturing, and coma; in infants with partial enzyme deficiencies, the symptoms may be delayed for months or years, the symptoms are more subtle, the hyperammonemia is less severe, and ammonia accumulation can be triggered by illness or stress throughout life.

E. Metabolic genetic disorders involving the urea cycle pathway include:
  1. **Ornithine transcarbamylase (OTC) deficiency.**
     a. OTC deficiency is an X-linked recessive genetic disorder caused by a mutation in the *OTC* gene on **chromosome Xp21.1** for **ornithine transcarbamylase.**
     b. OTC deficiency along with carbamoyl phosphate synthetase (CPSI) deficiency and N-acetyl glutamate synthetase (NAGS) deficiency are the most severe types of urea cycle disorders. Newborns with OTC deficiency rapidly develop hyperammonemia, and these children are always at risk for repeated bouts of hyperammonemia.
     c. OTC can be distinguished from CPSI deficiency by elevated levels of **orotic acid** in OTC individuals.
     d. Nearly 15% of female carriers develop hyperammonemia during their lifetime, and many require chronic medical management.
     e. **In the case of a male proband**, the father is not affected and is not a carrier because OTC deficiency males usually are sterile. The mother may be a carrier or the male proband may have a *de novo* mutation. The risk to the siblings of the male proband is 50% if the mother is a carrier. The risk to the siblings of the male proband is very low if the mother is not a carrier but greater than that of the general population since the possibility of germ line mosaicism exists. If the father has OTC deficiency, the chances of having any children is very low because OTC deficiency males usually are sterile. In the few fertile OTC deficiency males, the risk to all of his daughters is 100% and the risk to all of his sons is 0%.
     f. **In the case of a female proband**, the father or the mother may have transmitted the OTC mutation, or a de novo mutation may have occurred. The risk to the siblings of the female proband is 50% for her sisters and brothers if the mother is the carrier and 100% for her sisters and 0% for her brothers if the father is the carrier. If the mother has OTC deficiency, the risk to all of her children is 50% (her daughters will have a range of phenotypes, and her sons will be affected).
  2. **Other urea cycle disorders.** These include: CPSI deficiency, argininosuccinic acid synthetase (ASS) deficiency (or citrullinemia type I), argininosuccinic acid lyase (ASL) deficiency (or argininosuccinic aciduria), arginase (ARG) deficiency (or hyperargininemia), and NAGS deficiency.

Metabolic Genetic Disorders Involving Transport Pathways (Table 14-4)

A. MENKES DISEASE (MND).

1. MND is an X-linked recessive genetic disorder caused by various mutations in the *ATP7A* gene on **chromosome Xq12-q13** for **copper-transporting ATPase 1**, which is a P-type ATPase that transports copper across cell membranes, thereby controlling copper homeostasis.

2. MND is caused by small insertion and deletion mutations (35%), nonsense mutations (20%), RNA splicing mutations (15%), and missense mutations (8%).

3. These mutations result in low serum concentration of copper (0–60 ug/dL vs. 70–150 ug/dL normal), low serum concentration of ceruloplasmin (30–150 mg/dL vs. 200–450 mg/dL normal), a decreased intestinal absorption of copper, an accumulation of copper in some tissues, and a decreased activity of copper-dependent enzymes (e.g., dopamine β-hydroxylase critical for catecholamine synthesis or lysyl oxidase).

4. **In the case of a male proband**, the father is not affected and is not a carrier (MND males are sterile). The mother may be a carrier or the male proband may have a de novo mutation (≈30% of MND cases are simplex cases with no known family history). The risk to the siblings of the male proband is 50% if the mother is a carrier. The risk to the siblings of the male proband is very low if the mother is not a carrier but greater than that of the general population since the possibility of germ line mosaicism exists.

5. **In the case of a female proband**, the mother transmits the MND mutation, or a de novo mutation may have occurred. The risk to the siblings of the female proband is 50% for her sisters and brothers if the mother is a carrier. If the mother has MND, the risk to all of her children is 100% (her daughters will have a range of phenotypes, and her sons will be affected).

6. **Clinical features include**: infants initially appear normal up to 2–3 months of age but then develop hypotonia, seizures, failure to thrive, loss of developmental milestones, changes in hair (short, coarse, twisted, lightly pigmented, "steel wool" appearance), jowly facial appearance with sagging cheeks, temperature instability, hypoglycemia, urinary bladder diverticulae, and gastric polyps. Without early treatment with parenteral copper, MND progresses to severe neurodegeneration and death by 7 months–3 years of age.

B. WILSON DISEASE (WND).

1. WND is an autosomal recessive genetic disorder caused by >260 mutations in the *ATP7B* gene on chromosome **13q14.3-q21.1** for **copper-transporting ATPase 2**, which is a P-type ATPase expressed mainly in the kidney and liver that plays a key role in incorporating copper into ceruloplasmin and in the release of copper into bile.

2. WND is caused by either a missense mutation that results in a **normal histidine → glutamine** substitution at position 1069 (H1069Q), a missense mutation that results in a **normal arginine → leucine** substitution at position 778 (R778L), or a **15–base pair (bp) deletion** in the promoter region.

3. The H1069Q mutation accounts for 45% of cases in the European population. The R778L mutation accounts for 60% of cases in the Asian population. The 15-bp deletion mutation is common in the Sardinian population.

4. These mutations result in high hepatic concentration of copper (>250 ug/g dry weight vs. <55 ug/g dry weight normal), high urinary excretion of copper

($>$0.6 umol/24 hours), and damage of various tissues due to excessive accumulation of copper.

5. **Clinical features include**: symptoms occurring in individuals from 3–50 years of age, recurrent jaundice, hepatitislike illness, fulminant hepatic failure, tremors, poor coordination, loss of fine motor control, chorea, masklike facies, rigidity, gait disturbance, depression, neurotic behaviors, Kayser-Fleischer rings (deposition of copper in Descemet's membrane of the cornea), blue lunulae of the fingernails, and a high degree of copper storage in the body.

C. **HFE-ASSOCIATED HEREDITARY HEMOCHROMATOSIS (HHH).**

1. HHH is an autosomal recessive genetic disorder caused by $\approx$28 different mutations in the *HFE* gene on **chromosome 6p21.3** for **hereditary hemochromatosis protein**, which is a cell surface protein expressed as a heterodimer with ß$_2$-microglobulin, binds the transferrin receptor 1, and reduces cellular iron uptake, although the exact mechanism is unknown.

2. HHH is most commonly caused by two missense mutations that result in a **normal cysteine $\rightarrow$ tyrosine** substitution at position 282 (C282Y) resulting in decreased cell surface expression or in a **normal histidine $\rightarrow$ asparagine** substitution at position 63 (H63D) resulting in pH changes that affect binding to the transferrin receptor 1.

3. Nearly 87% of HHH-affected individuals in the European population are homozygous for the C282Y mutation or are **compound heterozygous** (i.e., two different mutations at the same gene locus) for the C282Y and H63D mutations.

4. These mutations result in elevated transferrin-iron saturation, elevated serum ferritin concentration, and hepatic iron overload assessed by Prussian blue staining of a liver biopsy.

5. If a person who has HHH decides to have a child, then the carrier risk factor becomes important. The risk that a partner of European descent is a heterozygote (Hh) is 11% (1 in 9 individuals) due the high carrier rate in the general European population for HHH.

6. **Clinical features include**: excessive storage of iron in the liver, heart, skin, pancreas, joints, and testes as well as abdominal pain, weakness, lethargy, weight loss, and hepatic fibrosis; without therapy, symptoms appear in males between 40 and 60 years of age and in females after menopause.

VI Metabolic Genetic Disorders Involving Degradation Pathways (Table 14-5)

Most complex biomolecules are recycled by degradation into simpler molecules, which then can be eliminated or used to synthesize new molecules. Malfunctions in degradation pathways will result in the accumulation (or "storage") of complex biomolecules within the cell. For example, lysosomal enzymes catalyze the stepwise degradation of glycosaminoglycans (GAGs; formerly called *mucopolysaccharides*), sphingolipids, glycoproteins, and glycolipids. **Lysosomal storage disorders (or mucopolysaccharidoses)** are caused by lysosomal enzyme deficiencies required for the stepwise degradation of GAGs that result in the accumulation of partially degraded GAGs within the cell leading to organ dysfunction.

A. **MUCOPOLYSACCHARIDOSIS TYPE I (MPS I).**

1. MPS I is an autosomal recessive genetic disorder caused by $\approx$57 different mutations in the *IDUA* gene on **chromosome 4p16.3** for **α-L-iduronidase**, which catalyzes the reaction that removes α-L-iduronate residues from heparan sulfate and dermatan sulphate during lysosomal degradation.

2. MPS I is the prototypical mucopolysaccharidoses disorder. MPS I presents as a continuum from severe to mild clinical symptoms, and MPS I–affected individuals are best described as having either **severe symptoms (MPS IH; Hurler syndrome)**, **intermediate symptoms (MPS IH/S; Hurler-Scheie syndrome)**, or **mild symptoms (MPS IS; Scheie syndrome)**.

3. MPS IH (Hurler syndrome) is most commonly caused by two nonsense mutations that result in a **normal tryptophan→nonsense** substitution at position 402 (W402X) or in a **normal glutamine→nonsense** substitution at position 70 (Q70X).

4. The W402X mutation accounts for 55% of cases in the Australasian population. The Q70X mutation accounts for 65% of cases in the Scandinavian population.

5. These mutations result in elevated heparan sulphate and dermatan sulphate excretion in the urine, reduced/absent α-L-iduronidase activity, and **heparan sulfate and dermatan sulfate** accumulation.

6. **Clinical features of MPS IH (Hurler syndrome) include**: infants initially appearing normal up to ≈9 months of age but then developing symptoms such as coarsening of facial features, thickening of alae nasi, lips, ear lobules, and tongue; corneal clouding; severe visual impairment; progressive thickening heart valves leading to mitral and aortic regurgitation; dorsolumbar kyphosis; skeletal dysplasia involving all of the bones; linear growth ceasing by 3 years of age; hearing loss; chronic recurrent rhinitis; severe mental retardation; and zebra bodies within neurons.

B. GAUCHER DISEASE (GD).

1. GD is an autosomal recessive genetic disorder caused by mutations in the *GBA* gene on **chromosome 1q21** for **β-glucosylceramidase**, which hydrolyzes glucocerebroside into glucose and ceramide.

2. GD is the most common lysosomal storage disorder. It presents as a continuum of clinical symptoms and is divided into three major clinical types (**types 1, 2, and 3**), which is useful in determining prognosis and management of the individual.

3. GD is most commonly caused by either a missense mutation that results in a **normal asparagine→serine** substitution at position 370 (N370S), a missense mutation that results in a **normal leucine→proline** substitution at position 444 (L444P), a 84GG mutation, or an IVS2+1 mutation.

4. The N370S, L444P, 84GG, and IVS2+1 mutations account for 95% of cases in the Ashkenazi Jewish population. These mutations result in absent/near absent β-glucosylceramidase activity and **glucosylceramide (and other glycolipids)** accumulation.

5. If one parent has GD (gg), the risk that a partner of Ashkenazi Jewish descent is a heterozygote is ≈5% (1 out of 18 individuals) due the high carrier rate in the general Ashkenazi Jewish population.

6. **Clinical features of type I GD include**: bone disease (e.g., focal lytic lesions, sclerotic lesions, osteonecrosis), which is the most debilitating pathology of type I GD; hepatomegaly; splenomegaly; cytopenia and anemia due to hypersplenism, splenic sequestration, and decreased erythropoiesis; and pulmonary disease (e.g., interstitial lung disease, alveolar/lobar consolidation; pulmonary hypertension). There is no primary central nervous system (CNS) involvement.

C. HEXOSAMINIDASE A DEFICIENCY (HAD).

1. **Acute infantile HAD (Tay-Sachs disease [TSD])** is the prototypical HAD. HAD presents as a group of neurodegenerative disorders caused by lysosomal accumulation of **GM2 ganglioside**.

2. TSD is an autosomal recessive genetic disorder caused by mutations in the *HEXA* gene on **chromosome 15q23-q24** for the **hexosaminidase α-subunit**, which

catalyzes the reaction that cleaves the terminal β-linked N-acetylgalactosamine from GM2 ganglioside.

3. TSD is most commonly caused by either a **4-bp insertion in exon 11 mutation** (+TATC1278) that produces a frameshift and a premature STOP codon or a **RNA splicing mutation in intron 12** (+1IVS12) that produces unstable messenger RNAs that are probably rapidly degraded.

4. The +TATC1278 and the +1IVS12 mutations account for ≈95% of cases in the Ashkenazi Jewish population. These mutations result in absent/near absent hexosaminidase A activity and **GM2 ganglioside** accumulation.

5. **Clinical features of TDS include**: infants initially appearing normal up to 3–6 months of age but then developing symptoms such as progressive weakness and loss of motor skills; decreased attentiveness; increased startled response; a cherry red spot in the fovea centralis of the retina; generalized muscular hypotonia; and later, progressive neurodegeneration, seizures, blindness, and spasticity followed by death at ≈2–4 years of age.

D. **OTHER GENETIC DISORDERS INVOLVING DEGRADATION PATHWAYS.** These include: mucopolysaccharidosis type II (MPS II; Hunter syndrome), mucopolysaccharidosis type IIIA (MPS IIIA; Sanfilippo A syndrome), mucopolysaccharidosis type IVA (MPS IVA; Morquio A syndrome), Niemann-Pick (NP) type 1A disorder, Fabry disorder, Krabbe disorder, and metachromatic leukodystrophy (MLD).

VII Summary Tables of Metabolic Genetic Disorders (Tables 14-1–14-5)

VIII Selected Photographs of Metabolic Genetic Disorders (Figure 14-1)

TABLE 14-1	METABOLIC GENETIC DISORDERS INVOLVING CARBOHYDRATE PATHWAYS	
Genetic Disorder	Gene/Gene Product Chromosome	Clinical Features
Galactosemia	*GALT* gene/galactose-1-phosphate uridylyltransferase 9p13	Feeding problems in the newborn, failure to thrive, hypoglycemia, hepatocellular damage, bleeding diathesis, jaundice, and hyperammonemia. Sepsis with *E. coli*, shock, and death may occur if the galactosemia is not treated.
Asymptomatic fructosuria	*KHK* gene/ketohexokinase or fructokinase 2p23.3-23.2	Presence of fructose in the urine
Hereditary fructose intolerance	*ALDOB* gene/ fructose 1-phosphate aldolase B 9q21.3-q22.2	Failure to thrive, fructosuria, hepatomegaly, jaundice, aminoaciduria, metabolic acidosis, lactic acidosis, low urine ketones, recurrent hypoglycemia and vomiting at the age of weaning when fructose or sucrose (a disaccharide that is hydrolyzed to glucose and fructose) is added to the diet;

(continued)

TABLE 14-1	METABOLIC GENETIC DISORDERS INVOLVING CARBOHYDRATE PATHWAYS *(Continued)*	
Genetic Disorder	**Gene/Gene Product Chromosome**	**Clinical Features**
		Infants and adults are asymptomatic until they ingest fructose or sucrose.
Lactose intolerance	*LCT* gene/lactase-phlorizin hydrolase 2q21	Diarrhea, crampy abdominal pain localized to the periumbilical area or lower quadrant; flatulence; nausea; vomiting; audible borborygmi; stools that are bulky, frothy, and watery; and bloating after milk or lactose consumption
GSD type Ia; von Gierke	*G6PC* gene/glucose-6-phosphatase 17q21	Accumulation of glycogen and fat in the liver and kidney resulting in hepatomegaly and renomegaly, severe hypoglycemia, lactic acidosis, hyperuricemia, hyperlipidemia, hypoglycemic seizures, doll-like faces with fat cheeks, relatively thin extremities, short stature, protuberant abdomen, and neutropenia with recurrent bacterial infections.
GSD type Ib; von Gierke	*SLC37A4* gene/glucose-6-phosphate translocase 11q23	
GSD type V; McArdle	*PYGM* gene/muscle glycogen phosphorylase 11q13	Exercise-induced muscle cramps and pain, "second wind" phenomenon with relief of myalgia and fatigue after a few minutes of rest, episodes of myoglobinuria, increased resting basal serum CK activity, onset typically occurring around 20–30 years of age; in preadolescents, clumsiness, lethargy, slow movement, and laziness
GSD type II; Pompe	*GAA* gene/lysosomal acid a-glucosidase 17q25.2-q25.3	Muscle and heart are affected.
GSD type IIIa; Cori	*AGL* gene/amylo-1,6glucosidase, 4-a-glucanotransferase (or glycogen branching enzyme) 1p21	Muscle and liver are affected.
GSD type IV; Andersen	*GBE1* gene/glucan(1,4-a-) branching enzyme 1 (or glycogen branching enzyme) 3	Muscle and liver are affected.
GSD type VI; Hers	*PYGL* gene/liver glycogen phosphorylase 14q11.2-q24.3	Liver is affected.
GSD type VII; Tarui	*PFKM* gene/muscle phosphofructokinase 12q13.11	Muscle is affected.

GSD, glycogen storage disease; CK, creatine kinase.

TABLE 14-2	METABOLIC GENETIC DISORDERS INVOLVING AMINO ACID PATHWAYS	
Genetic Disorder	**Gene/Gene Product Chromosome**	**Clinical Features**
Phenylalanine hydrolase deficiency (classic PKU)	*PAH* gene/phenylalanine hydrolase 12q23.2	No physical signs are apparent in neonates with PAH deficiency; diagnosis is based on detection of elevated plasma PAH concentration ($>$1,000 umol/L for classic PKU) and normal BH_4 cofactor metabolism; a dietary phenylalanine tolerance of $<$500 mg/day; untreated children with classic PKU show impaired brain development, microcephaly, epilepsy, severe mental retardation, behavioral problems, depression, anxiety, musty body odor, and skin conditions like eczema.
Hereditary tyrosinemia type I	*FAH* gene/fumarylacetoacetate hydrolase 15q23-q25	Diagnosis is based on detection of elevated plasma succinylacetone concentration, elevated plasma tyrosine, methionine, and phenylalanine concentrations; elevated urinary tyrosine metabolite (e.g., hydroxyphenylpyruvate) concentration, elevated urinary δ-aminolevulinic acid; cabbagelike odor; untreated children with HTI show severe liver dysfunction, renal tubular dysfunction, growth failure, and rickets.
Maple syrup disease	*BCKDHA* gene/E1a subunit of branched-chain ketoacid dehydrogenase complex (BCKD) 19q13.1-q13.2 *BCKDHB* gene/E1β subunit of BCKD 6q14 *DBT* gene/E2 subunit of BCKD 1p31	Untreated children with MSUD show maple syrup odor in cerumen 12–24 hours after birth; elevated plasma branched-chain amino acid concentration; ketonuria; irritability; poor feeding by 2–3 days of age; deepening encephalopathy including lethargy, intermittent apnea, opisthotonus, and stereotyped movements like "fencing" and "bicycling" by 4–5 days of age; acute leucine intoxication (leucinosis) associated with neurologic deterioration due to the ability of leucine to interfere with the transport of other large neutral amino acids across the blood–brain barrier, thereby reducing the amino acid supply to the brain.

PKU, phenylketonuria; MSUD, maple syrup urine disease.

TABLE 14-3	METABOLIC GENETIC DISORDERS INVOLVING THE UREA CYCLE PATHWAY	

Genetic Disorder	Gene/Gene Product Chromosome	Clinical Features
Ornithine transcarbamylase deficiency	*OTC* gene/ornithine transcarbamylase Xp21.1	Infants initially appear normal but then rapidly develop hyperammone- mia, cerebral edema, lethargy, anorexia, hyperventilation or hypoventilation, hypothermia, seizures, neurologic posturing, and coma; in infants with partial enzyme deficiencies, the symptoms may be delayed for months or years, the symptoms are more subtle, the hyperammonemia is less severe, and ammonia accumulation can be triggered by illness or stress throughout life.
Carbamoyl phosphate synthetase I deficiency	*CPS1* gene/carbamoylphosphate synthetase 1 2q35	
Argininosuccinic acid synthetase deficiency (or citrullinemia type I)	*ASS* gene/argininosuccinic acid synthetase 9q34	
Argininosuccinic acid lyase deficiency (or argininosuccinic aciduria)	*ASL* gene/argininosuccinic acid lyase 7cen-q11.2	
Arginase deficiency (or hyperargininemia)	*ARG1* gene/arginase 6q23	OTC deficiency and CPSI deficiency are the most severe types of urea cycle disorders.
N-acetyl glutamine synthetase deficiency	*NAGS* gene/N-acetyl glutamate synthetase 17q21.3	

OTC, ornithine transcarbamylase; CPSI, carbamoyl phosphate synthetase I.

TABLE 14-4	METABOLIC GENETIC DISORDERS INVOLVING TRANSPORT PATHWAYS	

Genetic Disorder	Gene/Gene Product Chromosome	Clinical Features
Menkes disease	*ATP7A* gene/copper-transporting ATPase 1 Xq12-q1	Infants initially appear normal up to 2–3 months of age but then develop hypotonia, seizures, failure to thrive, loss of developmental milestones, changes in hair (short, coarse, twisted, lightly pigmented, "steel wool" appearance), jowly facial appearance with sagging cheeks, temperature instability, hypoglycemia, urinary bladder diverticula, and gastric polyps. Without early treatment with par- enteral copper, MND progresses to severe neurodegeneration and death by 7 months–3 years of age.
Wilson disease	*ATP7B* gene/copper transporting ATPase 2 13q14.3-q21.1	Symptoms occur in individuals from 3–50 years of age, such as recur- rent jaundice, hepatitislike illness, fulminant hepatic failure, tremors, poor coordination, loss of fine

(continued)

| TABLE 14-4 | METABOLIC GENETIC DISORDERS INVOLVING TRANSPORT PATHWAYS *(Continued)* |

Genetic Disorder	Gene/Gene Product Chromosome	Clinical Features
		motor control, chorea, masklike facies, rigidity, gait disturbance, depression, neurotic behaviors, Kayser-Fleischer rings (deposition of copper in Descemet's membrane of the cornea), blue lunulae of the fingernails, and a high degree of copper storage in the body
HFE-associated hereditary hemochromatosis	*HFE* gene/hereditary hemochromatosis protein 6p21.3	Excessive storage of iron in the liver, heart, skin, pancreas, joints, and testes as well as abdominal pain, weakness, lethargy, weight loss, and hepatic fibrosis. Without therapy, symptoms appear in males between 40–60 years of age and in females after menopause.

MND, Menkes disease.

| TABLE 14-5 | METABOLIC GENETIC DISORDERS INVOLVING DEGRADATION PATHWAYS |

Genetic Disorder	Gene/Gene Product Chromosome	Accumulation Product	Clinical Features
Mucopolysaccharidosis type I (Hurler, Hurler-Scheie, or Scheie syndromes)	*IDUA* gene/a-L-iduronidase 4p16.3	Heparan sulfate Dermatan sulfate	Infants initially appearing normal up to ≈9 months of age but then developing symptoms such as coarsening of facial features, thickening of alae nasi, lips, ear lobules, and tongue; corneal clouding; severe visual impairment; progressive thickening heart valves leading to mitral and aortic regurgitation; dorsolumbar kyphosis; skeletal dysplasia involving all of the bones; linear growth ceasing by 3 years of age; hearing loss; chronic recurrent rhinitis; severe mental retardation; and zebra bodies within neurons.
Gaucher disease	*GBA* gene/ß-glucosylceramidase 1p21	Glucosylceramide Other glycolipids	Bone disease (e.g., focal lytic lesions, sclerotic lesions, osteonecrosis) is the most debilitating

(continued)

| TABLE 14-5 | METABOLIC GENETIC DISORDERS INVOLVING DEGRADATION PATHWAYS *(Continued)* |

Genetic Disorder	Gene/Gene Product Chromosome	Accumulation Product	Clinical Features
			pathology of type I GD; hepatomegaly; splenomegaly; cytopenia and anemia due to hyper-splenism, splenic seques-tration, and decreased erythropoiesis; and pulmonary disease (e.g., interstitial lung disease, alveolar/lobar consolidation; pulmonary hypertension). There is no primary CNS involvement.
Hexosaminidase A deficiency (Tay-Sachs)	*HEXA* gene/ hexosaminidase a-subunit 15q23-q24	GM2 ganglioside	Infants initially appearing normal up to 3–6 months of age but then developing symptoms such as progressive weakness and loss of motor skills; decreased attentiveness; increased startled response; a cherry red spot in the fovea centralis of the retina; generalized muscular hypotonia; and later, progressive neurode-generation, seizures, blind-ness, and spasticity followed by death at ≈2–4 years of age
Mucopolysaccharidosis type II (Hunter syndrome)	*IDS* gene/ iduronate 2-sulfatase Xq27.3-q28	Heparan sulfate Dermatan sulfate	Dysostosis multiplex (thickened skull, anterior thickening of ribs, vertebral abnormalities, and short/thick long bones), coarse face, hepatosplenomegaly, men-tal retardation, and behav-ioral problems
Mucopolysaccharidosis type III A(Sanfilippo A syndrome)	*SGSH* gene/ sulfamidase 17q25.3	Heparan sulfate	Dysostosis multiplex (thickened skull, anterior thickening of ribs, vertebral abnormalities, and short/thick long bones), mental retardation, and behavioral problems (aggressive behavior followed by progressive neurologic decline)

TABLE 14-5	**METABOLIC GENETIC DISORDERS INVOLVING DEGRADATION PATHWAYS** *(Continued)*		
Genetic Disorder	**Gene/Gene Product Chromosome**	**Accumulation Product**	**Clinical Features**
Mucopolysaccharidosis type IV A (Morquio A syndrome)	*GALNS* gene/ N-acetylgalac-tosamine-6-sulfate sulfatase 16q24.3	Keratan sulfate Chondroitin-6-sulfate	Short stature, bony dysplasia, and hearing loss
Niemann-Pick type 1A disorder	*SMPD1* gene/acid sphingomyeli-nase 11p15	Sphingomyelin	Hepatosplenomegaly, feeding difficulties, and loss of motor skills are seen between 1–3 months of age; a cherry red spot in the fovea centralis of the retina; and later, a rapid, profound, and progressive neurodegeneration followed by death at ≈2–3 years of age
Fabry disorder	*GLA* gene/a-galactosidase A Xq22	Globotriaosylce-ramide	In classically affected males, symptoms begin in child-hood or adolescence; such as severe neuropathic or limb pain precipitated by stress, extreme heat or cold, and physical exertion; telangiectasias, angiokeratomas in the groin, hip, and periumbili-cal regions; asymptomatic corneal deposits; retinal vascular tortuosity; in adult-hood, end-stage renal dis-ease, cardiac involvement, and cerebrovascular involvement leading to transient ischemic attacks and strokes.
Krabbe disorder	*GALC* gene/ galactocere-brosidase 14q31	Galactosylceramide	Developmental delay, limb stiffness, hypotonia, absent reflexes, optic atrophy, microcephaly, and extreme irritability between 1–6 months of age; later, seizures and tonic extensor spasms associated with light, sound, or touch stimulation occur; a rapid regression to the decere-brate condition followed by death at ≈2 years of age

(continued)

TABLE 14-5	METABOLIC GENETIC DISORDERS INVOLVING DEGRADATION PATHWAYS *(Continued)*		
Genetic Disorder	**Gene/Gene Product Chromosome**	**Accumulation Product**	**Clinical Features**
Metachromatic leukodystrophy	*ARSA* gene/ arylsulfatase A 22q13.3-qter	Cerebroside sulfate	Regression of motor skills, gait difficulties, ataxia, hypotonia, extensor plantar responses, and optic atrophy between 6 months and 2 years of age; later, peripheral neuropathy followed by death at ≈5–6 years of age

GD, Gaucher disease; CNS, central nervous system.

● **Figure14-1 Glycogen storage disease type I (von Gierke) (A1–A3). A1:** A 13-year-old boy with von Gierke disease. Note the enlarged abdomen. **A2:** Light micrograph of a liver biopsy shows hepatocytes with a pale, clear cytoplasm due to the large amount of accumulated glycogen that is extracted during histologic processing. **A3:** Electron micrograph of a liver biopsy shows hepatocytes filled with glycogen aggregates. **B: Glycogen storage disease type V (McArdle).** Light micrograph of a skeletal muscle biopsy shows muscle cells with a pale, clear cytoplasm due to the large amount of accumulated glycogen that is extracted during histologic processing. **C: Maple syrup urine disease.** T2-weighted magnetic resonance image shows hyperdensity in the brainstem *(arrows)*, indicating neurologic deterioration. **D: Wilson disease.** A Kayser-Fleischer ring *(arrows)* that is caused by the deposition of copper in the Descemet membrane and thereby obstructs the view of the underlying iris. **E: Hemochromatosis.** Light micrograph of a liver biopsy stained with Prussian blue shows hepatocytes with a heavily stained cytoplasm to the large amounts of accumulated iron. **F: Mucopolysaccharidosis type I (MPS I; Hurler syndrome).** An infant with coarsening of facial features; thickening of alae nasi, lips, ear lobules, and tongue; dorsolumbar kyphosis; and skeletal dysplasia involving all the bones. **G: Gaucher disease.** Light micrograph of a bone marrow aspirate smear shows the typical Gaucher cells with an abundant cytoplasm filled with fibrillarlike material. **H: Tay-Sachs disease.** Electron micrograph shows CNS neuron-filled lysosomes *(Lys)* containing whorls of membranelike material due to the large amounts of accumulated GM2 ganglioside. (N, nucleus of neuron.)

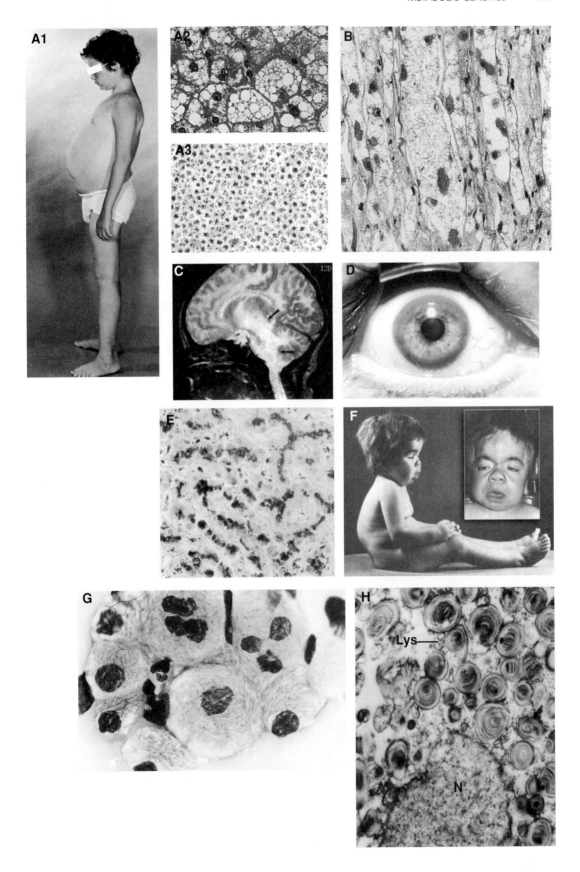

Chapter 15

Genetic Testing

Genetic Screening. *Genetic screening* is the "search in a population for persons possessing certain genotypes that: (1) are already associated with disease or predisposed to disease, or (2) may lead to disease in their descendants" (National Academy of Sciences, 1975). Genetic screening is a term used for genetic testing of a population in order to detect those at high risk.

A. **Genetic screening of newborns** is performed in all 50 U.S. states, but not all U.S. states perform the same tests. **Phenylketonuria, galactosemia, and congenital hypothyroidism** are screened in all 50 U.S. states. **Hemoglobinopathies** (e.g., sickle cell disease, thalassemias) are screened in a majority of U.S. states.

B. **Genetic screening of families** is performed when there is a positive history of a genetic condition (e.g., a family that has had one or more members born with a chromosome abnormality for chromosomal rearrangements).

Principles of Genetic Screening

A. Genetic screening should screen for a disease that is serious, is relatively common, has an effective treatment, and can be diagnosed prenatally (in some cases).

B. Genetic screening should be relatively inexpensive, easy to perform, valid, and reliable.

C. Genetic screening should have the necessary resources for diagnosis and treatment readily available.

D. A genetic screening test must have the appropriate sensitivity and specificity.
   1. **Sensitivity** is the ability to identify those **with the disease in question** measured as the proportion of **true positives**.
   2. **Specificity** is the ability to identify those **without the disease in question** measured as the proportion of **true negatives**.

Types of Genetic Screening

A. **PRENATAL GENETIC SCREENING.** Prenatal genetic screening for genetic disorders includes the following techniques:
   1. Fetal visualization.
   2. Population screening (e.g., maternal serum α-fetoprotein (MSAFP) triple screen).
   3. Amniocentesis.
   4. Chorionic villus sampling.
   5. Percutaneous umbilical blood sampling.

B. FAMILY GENETIC SCREENING. Family genetic screening for genetic disorders includes the following techniques:

1. Family history of a chromosomal rearrangement (e.g., translocation).
2. Genetic screening of female relatives in an X-linked pedigree (e.g., Duchenne muscular dystrophy).
3. Heterozygote screening in at-risk families (e.g., cystic fibrosis [CF]).
4. Presymptomatic screening (e.g., Huntington disease, breast cancer, colon cancer).

IV Some Examples of Genetic Screening

A. Tay-Sachs Disease.

1. Tay-Sachs disease is a severe autosomal recessive genetic disorder caused by a mutation in the *HEXA* gene on **chromosome 15q23-q24** for **hexosaminidase a-subunit** leading to the accumulation of GM2 ganglioside and neurodegeneration.
2. Tay-Sachs disease is especially prevalent in the Ashkenazi Jewish population. In this regard, the implementation of genetic screening programs and education in the Ashkenazi Jewish population have led to a **90% decline** in Tay-Sachs disease births.
3. Tay-Sachs disease has a 1 in 30 carrier frequency in the Ashkenazi Jewish population. Carrier testing can be done by using a biochemical assay (e.g., GM2 ganglioside) or by direct detection of *HEXA* gene mutations.
4. Options available to carrier couples are pregnancy termination and artificial insemination with noncarrier donors. In some Orthodox Jewish groups, carriers are forbidden to marry.

B. Thalassemias.

1. The thalassemias are a group of severe autosomal recessive genetic disorders caused by a lack of or decreased synthesis of either the hemoglobin α-chain (**α-thalassemia**) or the hemoglobin β-chain (**β-thalassemia**).

   a. **α-thalassemia.** α-thalassemia is an autosomal recessive genetic disorder caused by a mutation in the *HBA1* gene and the *HBA2* gene on **chromosome 16pter-p13.3** for the **hemoglobin α_1 chain** and **hemoglobin α_2 chain**, respectively.

      i. **Hb Bart hydrops fetalis (Hb Bart)** results from the deletion or dysfunction of all four α-globin alleles. Hb Bart is the most severe form of α-thalassemia. **Clinical features include:** fetal onset of generalized edema, ascites, pleural and pericardial effusions, and severe hypochromatic anemia.

      ii. **Hemoglobin H (HbH)** results from the deletion or dysfunction of three α-globin alleles. **Clinical features include:** mild microcytic hypochromatic hemolytic anemia and hepatosplenomegaly.

      iii. α^0**-thalassemia** results from the deletion or dysfunction of two α-globin alleles. This is a **carrier state** for α-thalassemia.

      iv. α^+**-thalassemia** results from the deletion or dysfunction of one α-globin alleles. This is a **carrier state** for α-thalassemia.

   b. **β-thalassemia major.** β-thalassemia major is an autosomal recessive genetic disorder caused by a mutation in the *HBB* gene on **chromosome 11p15.5** for the **hemoglobin β chain.** **β-thalassemia major** is the most severe form of β-thalassemia leading to a severe, transfusion-dependent anemia. The carrier state is often referred to as **β-thalassemia minor.**

2. α-thalassemia is prevalent in the Asian and African populations. β-thalassemia is prevalent in the Mediterranean population. The thalassemias are so common that many individuals carry several different mutations. In this regard, the implementation of genetic screening programs and education in the Mediterranean regions have led to a 75% **decline** in thalassemia disease births.

3. The thalassemias have a 1 in 30 carrier frequency in the Mediterranean population. Carrier testing can be done by using DNA sequencing, or if the mutation in a family is known, allele-specific oligonucleotide (ASO) testing for the specific mutation can be performed.

4. Because the disease is so severe, pregnancy termination is an acceptable option. In some areas of this region, carrier testing is required before marriage. Reproductive decisions may be aided by knowledge of disease status and can provide assurance to those who do not have the mutation.

C. CYSTIC FIBROSIS.

1. CF is an autosomal recessive genetic disorder caused by >1,000 mutations in the *CFTR* **gene** on **chromosome 7q31.2** for the **cystic fibrosis transmembrane conductance regulator,** which functions as a chloride ion (Cl⁻) channel.

2. The prevalence of CF is 1 in 3,200 in whites, 1 in 15,00 in blacks, and 1 in 31,000 in Asian Americans.

3. CF has a 1 in 28 carrier frequency in whites, 1 in 61 in blacks, and 1 in 29 in Ashkenazi Jews. Carrier testing can be done by using the ACMG pan-ethnic 23-mutation panel. CF carrier testing is recommended for non-Jewish whites and Ashkenazi Jews. CF carrier testing is also offered as routine prenatal care in some centers.

4. Prenatal genetic testing for pregnancies at 50% risk is available by DNA analysis of fetal cells obtained by amniocentesis (at ≈15–18 weeks of gestation) or chorionic villus sampling (at ≈12 weeks of gestation). *CFTR* gene mutations must be identified in both parents before prenatal testing can be done.

5. When *CFTR* gene mutations are identified in both parents, pregnancy can be achieved through assisted reproductive technology. In this case, preimplantation genetic testing is available by using embryonic cells obtained from a multicell stage embryo during the *in vitro* fertilization technique.

D. PRESYMPTOMATIC SCREENING.
Presymptomatic screening is available for Huntington disease, autosomal dominant breast cancer (BRCA1 and BRCA2), familial adenomatous polyposis coli (FAPC), hereditary nonpolyposis colorectal cancer (HNPCC), and hereditary hemochromatosis.

1. Huntington disease (HD).

a. HD is an autosomal dominant genetic disorder caused by a 36 → 100+ unstable repeat sequence of (CAG)ₙ located in the *HD* **gene** on **chromosome 4p16.3** for the **huntingtin** protein leading to movement jerkiness that is most apparent at movement termination, chorea (dancelike movements), memory deficits, affective disturbances, personality changes, and dementia. HD is protracted, invariably fatal, and has no treatment.

b. Asymptomatic at-risk adults seek genetic testing in order to make personal decisions regarding careers, financial estates, reproductive decisions, or just the "need to know." Reproductive decisions may be aided by knowledge of disease status and can provide assurance to those who do not have the mutation. Genetic testing of asymptomatic at-risk adults does not accurately predict the exact age of onset, severity, type of symptoms, or the rate of progression.

However, the size of the CAG trinucleotide repeat does generally correlate with age of onset. Extensive pre- and posttesting counseling is required to address issues such as disability insurance coverage, employment discrimination, educational discrimination, changes family interactions, depression, and suicide ideation.

    c. Genetic testing of asymptomatic at-risk individuals <18 years of age is generally not recommended.

    d. Prenatal genetic testing for pregnancies at 50% risk is available by DNA analysis of fetal cells obtained by amniocentesis (at $\approx$15–18 weeks of gestation) or chorionic villus sampling (at $\approx$12 weeks of gestation).

2. Autosomal dominant <u>br</u>east <u>c</u>ancer (BRCA1 and BRCA2).

    a. BRCA1 and BRCA2 are autosomal dominant genetic disorders caused by mutations in the *BRCA1* **gene** and *BRCA2* **gene** on **chromosomes 17q21 and 13q12.3**, respectively, for the **breast cancer type 1 susceptibility protein** and the **breast cancer type 2 susceptibility protein** leading to a predisposition to breast, ovarian, and prostate cancers.

    b. Genetic testing of asymptomatic at-risk adults and children can be used with certainty when a clinically diagnosed relative undergoes genetic testing and the specific mutation in the *BRCA1* or *BRCA2* gene is identified. In general, genetic testing of asymptomatic at-risk adults and children is not performed.

    c. When a clinically diagnosed relative is not available, failure to identify an BRCA1 or BRCA2 disease-causing mutation in the at-risk adult or child does not eliminate the possibility that a BRCA1 or BRCA2 disease-causing mutation is present in the at-risk adult or child.

    d. BRCA1 and BRCA2 genetic testing is expensive, as it involves sequencing all of the exons and some intron sequences. If BRCA1 and BRCA2 genetic testing reveals a high risk for breast cancer, there are unfortunately no surefire preventive measures available. In this regard, prophylactic removal of breasts (and ovaries) and chemoprevention by using tamoxifen only reduces the risk of breast cancer but does not eliminate it. However, these individuals may benefit from increased surveillance by using monthly breast self-examination, annual clinical breast examination, annual mammography, and breast magnetic resonance imaging, which can detect a tumor but not prevent it.

3. Familial adenomatous polyposis coli.

    a. FAPC is an autosomal dominant genetic disorder caused by a mutation in the *APC* **antioncogene (or tumor suppressor gene)** on **chromosome 5q21-q22** for the **APC protein** leading to the development of 500–2,000 polyps that carpet the mucosal surface of the colon and invariably become malignant. FAPC accounts for $\approx$1% of all colorectal cancer cases and involves a mutation in the *APC* **tumor suppressor gene**. The progression from a small polyp to a large polyp is associated with a mutation in the *ras* **proto-oncogene**. The progression from a large polyp to metastatic carcinoma is associated with mutations in the *DCC* **tumor suppressor gene** (deleted in colon carcinoma) and the *p53* **tumor suppressor gene**.

    b. Genetic testing of asymptomatic at-risk adults and children can be used with certainty when a clinically diagnosed relative undergoes genetic testing and the specific mutation in the *APC* gene is identified.

    c. When a clinically diagnosed relative is not available, failure to identify an APC disease-causing mutation in the at-risk adult or child does not eliminate the possibility that an APC disease-causing mutation is present in the at-risk adult or child.

d. Those with mutations for APC can benefit from early diagnosis. With regular monitoring by colonoscopy beginning at ≈10 years of age, polyps can be removed so that they cannot develop into malignancies.

e. Prenatal genetic testing for pregnancies at 50% risk is available by DNA analysis of fetal cells obtained by amniocentesis (at ≈15–18 weeks of gestation) or chorionic villus sampling (at ≈12 weeks of gestation). The APC disease-causing mutation in an affected family member must be identified before prenatal testing is performed.

4. Hereditary nonpolyposis colorectal cancer.

a. HNPCC is an autosomal dominant genetic disorder caused by mutations in the *MLH1, MSH2, MSH6,* and *PMS2* **genes** on chromosomes **3p21.3, 2p22-p21, 2p16,** and **7p22,** respectively, for various **DNA mismatch repair enzymes** leading to colorectal cancer. HNPCC accounts for 3%–5% of all colorectal cancers. HNPCC is characterized by: onset of colorectal cancer at a young age, high frequency of carcinomas proximal to the splenic flexure, multiple synchronous or metachronous colorectal cancers, and presence of extracolonic cancers (e.g., endometrial and ovarian cancer; adenocarcinomas of the stomach, small intestine, and hepatobiliary tract).

b. Genetic testing of asymptomatic at-risk adults and children can be used with certainty when a clinically diagnosed relative undergoes genetic testing and the specific mutation is identified. Genetic testing of asymptomatic at-risk adults and children does not accurately predict the exact age of onset, severity, type of symptoms, or the rate of progression.

c. When a clinically diagnosed relative is not available, failure to identify a disease-causing mutation in the at-risk adult or child does not eliminate the possibility that a disease-causing mutation is present in the at-risk adult or child.

d. Those with mutations in the *MLH1, MSH2, MSH6, PMS1,* and *PMS2* genes for HPNCC can benefit from early diagnosis. Genetic testing of asymptomatic at-risk individuals <18 years of age is generally not recommended. In rare cases, individuals have been diagnosed with HPNCC at very young ages, so some clinicians recommend that genetic screening begins 10 years before the earliest age of onset in the family. With regular monitoring by colonoscopy, polyps can be removed so that they cannot develop into malignancies.

e. Prenatal genetic testing for pregnancies at 50% risk is available by DNA analysis of fetal cells obtained by amniocentesis (at ≈15–18 weeks of gestation) or chorionic villus sampling (at ≈12 weeks of gestation). The specific disease-causing mutation in an affected family member must be identified before prenatal testing is performed.

5. Hereditary hemochromatosis (HH).

a. HH is an autosomal recessive genetic disorder caused by a mutation in the **HFE gene** on **chromosome 6p21.3** for the **hereditary hemochromatosis protein** leading to excessive accumulation of iron in the liver, pancreas, skin, heart, joints, and testes.

b. HH has a 1 in 8 carrier frequency in northern Europeans. Since the penetrance of the genotype is low and the natural outcome of untreated HH individuals cannot be predicted, no uniform recommendations for population screening have been adopted. Treatment is serial phlebotomy, which can give a normal life expectancy.

c. Prenatal genetic testing for pregnancies at increased risk is available by DNA analysis of fetal cells obtained by amniocentesis (at ≈15–18 weeks of gestation) or chorionic villus sampling (at ≈12 weeks of gestation). The specific disease-causing mutation in an affected family member must be identified before prenatal testing is performed. Prenatal genetic testing for HH is rarely requested.

Ⓥ Limitations of Genetic Testing

A. Genetic testing is never 100% accurate. For example, mosaicism can confound cytogenetic results even though the accuracy of the genetic test approaches 100%. In addition, human error is always a possibility.

B. Genetic testing cannot detect the presence of disease. For example, a genetic test for hereditary breast cancer cannot predict who will get the disease.

C. Genetic testing may not detect all of the mutations causing the disease. For example, autosomal dominant breast cancer, CF, and Marfan syndrome all have multiple mutations that may cause the disease. In general, it is not practical to test for all mutations.

D. Genetic testing can lead to complex ethical and social considerations, which include but are not limited to the following:
   1. Discrimination by employers or insurance companies.
   2. Lack of effective treatment for the condition (e.g., Huntington disease, familial Alzheimer disease).
   3. Results may affect family members who do not wish to know about their risk for a genetic disorder.
   4. Family members who are at risk for a genetic disorder may not wish to share this information with other family members.
   5. "Survivor guilt," where those who do not test positive for a mutated gene may feel guilty when others in the family do test positive.

Ⓥ Ⅰ Methods Used for Genetic Testing

A. SOUTHERN BLOTTING AND PRENATAL TESTING FOR SICKLE CELL ANEMIA. Southern blotting is a technique that provides a good example of the basic concepts used in genetic testing, although many other techniques have been developed and used in clinical testing laboratories. For example, many genetic testing laboratories use targeted mutational analysis via polymerase chain reaction for sickle cell anemia testing **(Figure 15-1).**

B. SANGER DNA SEQUENCING (Figure 15-2). DNA sequencing is used in genetic testing when a large number of different gene mutations are associated with the disease (e.g., those mutations in the *BRCA1* and *BRCA2* genes associated with breast cancer). Sanger DNA sequencing is limited by the number of nucleotides that can sequence at one time, so restriction enzymes are often used to digest the DNA into manageable chunks. This basic technique has been modified, and sequencing is now mostly automated. High throughput DNA sequencers using a different methodology are now available.

C. DOT BLOT HYBRIDIZATION USING ASOs (Figure 15-3). This genetic test is used for direct mutation detection in heterozygote screening (e.g., CF).

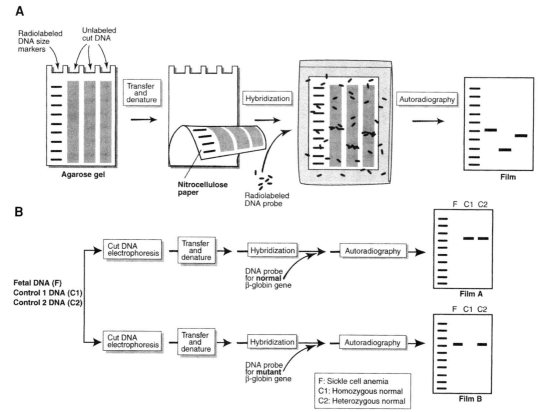

● **Figure 15-1 Southern blotting and prenatal testing for sickle cell anemia.** Southern blotting allows for the identification of a specific DNA sequence (e.g., gene for the β-globin chain of hemoglobin) by using a **DNA probe** and the **hybridization reaction.** A DNA probe is a single-stranded piece of DNA (10–120 base pair **oligonucleotide**) that participates in a hybridization reaction. A hybridization reaction is a reaction whereby a single-stranded piece of DNA (like a DNA probe) binds (or hybridizes) with another piece of single-stranded DNA of complementary nucleotide sequence. The hybridization reaction exploits a fundamental property of DNA to denature and renature. The two strands of double helix DNA are held together by **weak hydrogen bonds** that can be broken (denatured) by **high temperature** (90°C) or **alkaline pH** such that single-stranded DNA is formed. Under **low temperature** or **acid pH,** single-stranded DNA will reform double helix DNA (renature). **A: Southern blotting.** Double-stranded DNA is cut by three different restriction enzymes and separated by gel electrophoresis into three separate lanes. One lane is reserved for radiolabeled DNA size markers. The double-stranded DNA is transferred to a nitrocellulose paper under alkaline conditions so the DNA is denatured into single strands. The nitrocellulose paper is placed in a plastic bag along with the radiolabeled DNA probe and is incubated under conditions that favor hybridization. The nitrocellulose paper is exposed to photographic film (autoradiography) so that the radiolabeled probe will show up as bands. **B: Prenatal testing for sickle cell anemia.** It is good news when you hear that a gene has been cloned and sequenced, because now a DNA probe that hybridizes to the gene can be made and used, for example, in prenatal testing for sickle cell anemia. Sickle cell anemia is a recessive genetic disease caused by a mutation in the β-globin gene that results in a change of single amino acid from **glutamic acid** (normal) to **valine** (mutant) in the β-globin protein. Both the normal gene and mutant gene for β-globin protein have been sequenced so that DNA probes can be made to locate both of these genes in a Southern blot. Fetal DNA *(F)* is obtained from a high-risk fetus and compared with control DNA *(C1* and *C2)*. The DNA is separated into two samples. Each sample is cut with restriction enzymes, subjected to gel electrophoresis, and transferred to nitrocellulose paper under denaturing conditions. One sample is hybridized with a DNA probe for the normal β-globin gene, and the other sample is hybridized with a DNA probe for the mutant β-globin gene. After autoradiography, the films A and B can be analyzed. You will likely be asked to interpret a Southern blot on the USMLE for either an autosomal recessive, autosomal dominant, or X-linked genetic disease. Examine Lane F (fetal DNA) in films A and B. Note that Lane F has no bands in Film A (no normal β-globin gene) but has one band in Film B (mutant β-globin gene). This means that the fetus is homozygous for the mutant β-globin gene and therefore will have sickle cell anemia. Examine Lane C1 (control DNA) in films A and B. Note that Lane C1 has one band in Film A but no bands in Film B. This means that this person is homozygous for the normal β-globin gene and therefore will be normal. Examine Lane C2 (control DNA) in films A and B. Note that Lane C2 has one band in Film A and one band in Film B. This means that this person is heterozygous, having one copy of the normal β-globin gene and one copy of the mutant β-globin gene. This person will be normal since sickle cell anemia is genetic recessive disease, so two copies of the mutant β-globin gene are necessary for sickle cell anemia to appear.

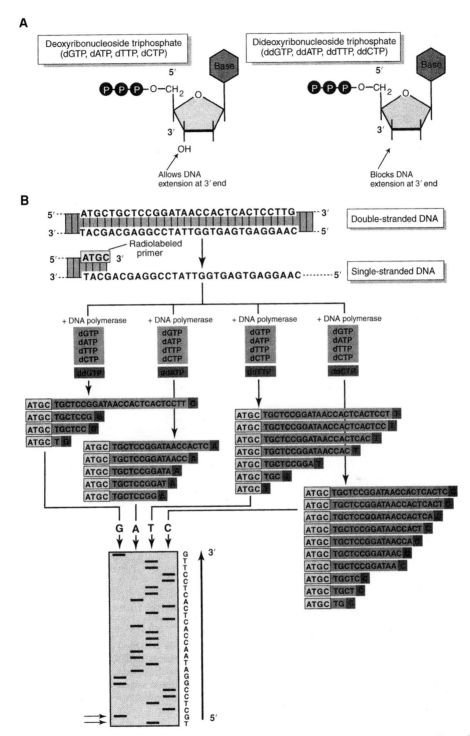

● **Figure 15-2 The enzymatic method of Sanger DNA sequencing.** Although restriction maps provide useful information concerning a DNA sample, the ultimate physical map of DNA is its **nucleotide sequence.** The nucleotide sequence is established by a technique called *DNA sequencing*. This method employs the use of DNA synthesis with **dideoxyribonucleoside triphosphates,** which **lack the 3'-OH group** that is normally found on deoxyribonucleoside triphosphates. If a dideoxyribonucleoside triphosphate becomes incorporated into DNA during synthesis, the addition of the next nucleotide is **blocked** due to the lack of the 3'-OH group. This forms the basis of the enzymatic method of DNA sequencing. **A:** The biochemical structure of deoxyribonucleoside triphosphates (dGTP, dATP, dTTP, dCTP) and dideoxyribonucleoside triphosphates (ddGTP, ddATP, ddTTP, ddCTP) is shown. Note the lack of the 3'-OH group on the dideoxyribonucleoside triphosphates. (*continued*)

● **Figure 15-2** *Continued*. **B:** Double-stranded DNA is separated into single strands, and one of the strands is used as the template. A radiolabeled primer (ATGC) is used to initiate DNA synthesis. Four separate reaction mixtures are set up, containing DNA polymerase, dGTP, dATP, dTTP, dCTP and **either** ddGTP, ddATP, ddTTP, ddCTP. These four reactions will produce a number of different-length DNA fragments that will terminate in either a G, A, T, or C depending on which dideoxyribonucleoside triphosphate was present in the reaction mixture. The contents of each reaction mixture is separated by gel electrophoresis based on size of the DNA fragments. The gel is then exposed to film such that the radiolabeled primer will identify each of the DNA fragments as bands. The bands are arranged as four parallel columns representing DNA fragments of varying lengths that terminate in either G, A, T, or C. A typical DNA sequencing film is shown, and you may be asked on the USMLE is read a sequencing gel. Start at the bottom the film and identify the lowest band (i.e., the shortest DNA fragment), and note that the lowest band in found in the T column (→). Now you know that the first nucleotide in the sequence is T. Go the next lowest band on the film, and note that it is found under the G column (→). Now you know that the second nucleotide in the sequence is G. Continue this process for all 26 bands. Please note that when you start at the bottom of the film and go up, you will be constructing the DNA sequence in a **5′→3′ direction.**

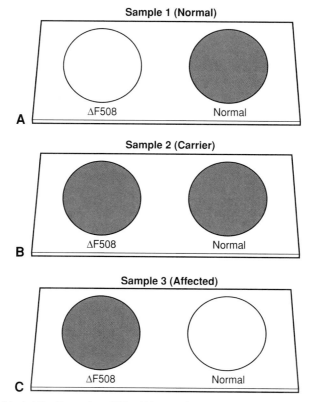

● **Figure 15-3 Dot blot hybridization using ASOs.** This genetic test involves taking an aqueous solution of target DNA from the patient (e.g., blood sample or epithelial swab). The denatured target DNA is spotted on a nitrocellulose membrane and allowed to dry. The denatured target DNA is now immobilized on the membrane and exposed to a solution containing a single-stranded labeled (P^{32} or immunofluorescence) ASO probe. An ASO probe distinguishes between alleles that differ by even a single nucleotide substitution. An ASO probe is typically 15–20 nucleotides long and is used under hybridization conditions where the DNA duplex between the target DNA and ASO probe is stable only if there is perfect base complementarity between them. **A:** Sample 1 (normal individual). The immobilized denatured target DNA is exposed to an ASO probe for either the deltaF508 mutation of the *CFTR* gene for CF or the normal *CFTR* gene for CF. In this case, the individual is negative for the deltaF508 mutation (*white circle*) and positive for the normal *CFTR* gene (*dark circle*). **B:** Sample 2 (carrier individual). The immobilized denatured target DNA is exposed to an ASO probe for either the deltaF508 mutation of the *CFTR* gene for CF or the normal *CFTR* gene for CF. In this case, the individual is positive for the deltaF508 mutation (*dark circle*) and positive for the normal *CFTR* gene (*dark circle*); hence, a heterozygote carrier. **C:** Sample 3 (affected individual). The immobilized denatured target DNA is exposed to an ASO probe for either the deltaF508 mutation of the *CFTR* gene for CF or the normal *CFTR* gene for CF. In this case, the individual is positive for the deltaF508 mutation (*dark circle*) and negative for the normal *CFTR* gene (*white circle*).

Chapter 16

Reproductive Risk Assessment

Ⅰ **Autosomal Dominant Inheritance.** In autosomal dominant disorders, males and females are equally affected, male-to-male transmission occurs, and multiple generations are affected.

A. Example 1: In autosomal dominant disorders, the affected parent is usually a heterozygote because homozygosity for an autosomal dominant allele is frequently a genetic lethal (where those with the disorder die before they reproduce). In this example, the father has the disorder caused by the autosomal dominant allele "D." All possible combinations of alleles from the parents are shown in the following Punnet square.

	Mother	
	d	d
Father		
D	Dd	Dd
d	dd	dd

Conclusion: There is a **50% chance** (2 out of 4 children) of having a child with the autosomal dominant disorder (Dd), assuming complete penetrance.

B. Example 2: In some autosomal dominant disorders (e.g., achondroplasia), it is not unusual for individuals to choose partners who have the same condition. The parents may actually be more concerned about the chances of having a child with normal stature than one with achondroplasia. As mentioned previously, homozygosity for an autosomal dominant allele is frequently a genetic lethal, so both parents with achondroplasia would be heterozygous. In this example, the father and the mother have the disorder caused by the autosomal dominant allele "A." All possible combinations of alleles from the parents are shown in the following Punnet square.

	Mother	
	A	a
Father		
A	AA	Aa
a	Aa	aa

Conclusion: There is a **50% chance** (2 out of 4 children) of having a child with achondroplasia (Aa), a **25% chance** (1 out of 4 children) of having a normal child (aa), and a **25% chance** (1 out of 4 children) of having a child with a lethal condition (AA).

C. **Example 3:** In some autosomal dominant disorders (e.g., Huntington disorder), homozygosity for an autosomal dominant allele is not a genetic lethal, so the affected individual would be homozygous. This situation is exceedingly rare and would most likely occur in cases of consanguinity, where the parents are related. In this example, the mother has the disorder caused by the autosomal dominant allele "H." All possible combinations of alleles from the parents are shown in the following Punnet square.

		Mother	
		H	H
Father			
h		Hh	Hh
h		Hh	Hh

Conclusion: There is a **100% chance** (4 out of 4 children) of having a child with Huntington disorder (Hh).

Autosomal Recessive Inheritance.

In autosomal recessive disorders, males and females are equally affected, and both parents must be carriers of a single copy of the responsible gene in order for the child to be affected unless there is a *de novo* mutation or uniparental disomy (see Chapter 6). In addition, consanguinity is always a possibility, especially if the condition is rare.

A. **Example 1:** In autosomal recessive disorders, both parents are carriers of a single copy of the responsible gene. In this example, the mother and father are heterozygous carriers of the autosomal recessive allele "r." All possible combinations of alleles from the parents are shown in the following Punnet square.

		Mother	
		R	r
Father			
R		RR	Rr
r		Rr	rr

Conclusion: There is a **25% chance** (1 out of 4 children) of having a child with the autosomal recessive disorder (rr), a **50% chance** (2 out of 4 children) of having a normal child that will be a heterozygous carrier (Rr), and a **25% chance** (1 out of 4 children) of having a normal child that will **NOT** be a carrier (RR).

B. **Example 2:** In autosomal recessive disorders, the genetic risk for the normal children being homozygous or heterozygous can be calculated. In this calculation, the child with the autosomal recessive disorder (rr = X) is eliminated from the calculation. In this example, the mother and father are heterozygous carriers of the autosomal recessive

allele "r." All possible combinations of alleles from the parents are shown in the following Punnet square.

	Mother	
	R	r
Father		
R	RR	Rr
r	Rr	X

Conclusion: There is a **66% chance** (2 out of 3 children) of having a normal child
that is a heterozygous carrier (Rr). There is a **33% chance** (1 out of 3 children) of having a normal child that is homozygous (RR).

X-Linked Recessive Inheritance. In X-linked recessive disorders, only males are
affected (affected females are rare), females are carriers, and there is no father-to-son transmission because the sons receive only the Y chromosome from the father.

A. **Example 1:** In this example, the mother is a carrier (X^aX) and the father is normal
    (XY). All possible combinations of alleles from the parents are shown in the following
    Punnet square.

	Mother	
	X^a	X
Father		
X	X^aX	XX
Y	X^aY	XY

Conclusion: There is a **50% chance** (1 out of 2 sons) of having a son with the X-linked
recessive disorder (X^aY). There is a **50% chance** (1 out of 2 daughters) of having a
daughter who is a carrier of the X-linked recessive allele (X^aX).

B. **Example 2:** In this example, the mother is normal (XX) and the father has the disor-
    der (X^aY). All possible combinations of alleles from the parents are shown in the fol-
    lowing Punnet square.

	Mother	
	X	X
Father		
X^a	X^aX	X^aX
Y	XY	XY

Conclusion: There is a **100% chance** (2 out of 2 daughters) of having a daughter who
is a carrier of the X-linked recessive allele (X^aX). There is a **100% chance** (2 out of 2
sons) of having a normal son (XY); that is, there in no father-to-son transmission.

C. Example 3: In this example, the mother is a carrier (X^aX) and the father has the disorder (X^aY). This may occur in rare cases (e.g., usually consanguineous unions). In addition, as treatment of affected males becomes more effective, the prevalence of affected males that live long enough and are healthy enough to reproduce is increasing. All possible combinations of alleles from the parents are shown in the following Punnet square.

		Mother	
		X^a	X
Father			
X^a		X^aX^a	X^aX
Y		X^aY	XY

Conclusion: There is a **50% chance** (1 out of 2 daughters) of having a daughter with the X-linked recessive disorder (X^aX^a); this is unusual in X-linked recessive disorders. There is **50% chance** (1 out of 2 daughters) of having a daughter who is a carrier of the X-linked recessive allele (X^aX). There is a **50% chance** (1 out of 2 sons) of having a son with the X-linked recessive disorder (X^aY). There is a **50% chance** (1 out of 2 sons) of having a normal son (XY).

D. Haldane's rule. If a male is conceived with an X-linked LETHAL condition and he is the only case in the family, there is a **66% chance** that his mother is a carrier of the X-linked recessive allele (X^aX). This risk is derived from a formula that takes into account the number of new mutations in the population for certain X-linked lethal disorders.

IV Consanguinity. Consanguinity is mating with someone to whom you are related.

A. Consanguinity is higher among parents of children with rare autosomal recessive diseases.

B. Consanguinity increases the incidence of multifactorial inherited disorders. The risk for birth defects is almost double the general population risk in first cousin matings.

C. Coefficient of relationship (COR). COR is the proportion of genes in common between two related individuals. COR is described by the equation below.

$$COR = (½)^{n-1}$$

where, n = number of individuals in the path.

D. Coefficient of inbreeding (COI) or homozygous by descent. COI is the probability that an individual is homozygous at a locus as a result of consanguinity in his or her parents. COI is described by the equation below.

$$COI = (COR)1/2$$

E. Summary table of COI (Table 16-1)

F. Example of consanguinity (Figure 16-1). Paula is a carrier of congenital Finnish nephrosis (CFN), a rare autosomal recessive kidney disease. If she mates with her first cousin Simon (a cousin through her maternal uncle), what is the chance that he also carries the abnormal gene?

TABLE 16-1	COEFFICIENT OF INBREEDING		
Relationship	Degree of Relationship	COR	COI
Parent–child	1st degree	½ (50%)	¼ (25%)
Siblings	1st degree	½ (50%)	¼ (25%)
Uncle–niece	2nd degree	¼ (25%)	⅛ (12%)
First cousins	3rd degree	⅛ (12%)	¹⁄₁₆ (6%)
Second cousins	5th degree	¹⁄₃₂ (3%)	¹⁄₆₄ (1.5%)

COR, coefficient of relationship; COI, coefficient of inbreeding.

1. **How many individuals are in the pedigree path?** Begin with Paula, and ascend the pedigree path to one of the common ancestors (in this example, it is Paula's grandfather). Then, descend the pedigree to Simon. Counting Paula and Simon, there are five individuals in this path (note the numbering on the pedigree). **Therefore, n = 5.**

2. **What is the COR between Paula and Simon through the grandfather and grandmother?**
   a. Calculate the COR between Paula and Simon through the grandfather: $COR = (1/2)^{n-1} = (1/2)^{5-1} = (1/2)^4 = 1/16 \ (6\%)$. Consequently, there is a 6% chance that Simon has inherited the gene if it was passed through the grandfather.
   b. Calculate the COR between Paula and Simon through the grandmother (because they also share their grandmother as a common ancestor, the COR must be calculated for her the same way): $COR = (1/2)^{n-1} = (1/2)^{5-1} = (1/2)^4 = 1/16 \ (6\%)$. Consequently, there is a 6% chance that Simon has inherited the gene if it was passed through the grandmother.
   c. Calculate the final COR for first cousins: Add the common ancestors' CORs: $1/16 + 1/16 = 1/8 \ (12\%)$. Therefore, the final COR for first cousins is 1/8 (12%). This can be interpreted as a **1/8 (12%)** chance that Simon is a carrier of the abnormal gene.

3. **If Paula and Simon have a child that is affected with CFN, what is the chance that the child inherited both abnormal alleles from a common ancestor?** The COR for first cousins is 1/8. So, $COI = (COR)\frac{1}{2} = (1/8)(1/2) = 1/16 \ (6\%)$. This can be interpreted as a **1/16 (6%)** chance that the CFN-affected child inherited both abnormal alleles from a common ancestor.

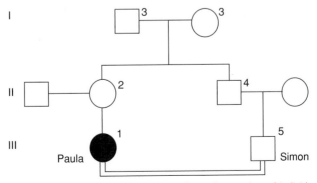

● **Figure 16-1 A pedigree of consanguinity.** The numbers indicate the number of individuals in the pedigree path, which can be counted through Paula's grandfather (3) or Paula's grandmother (3). In both cases, there are five individuals in the path.

Figure Credits

Figure 1-1: From Dudek RW. *HY Cell and Molecular Biology*, 2nd ed. Baltimore: Lippincott Williams & Wilkins, 2007:84, Figure 10-1.

Figure 1-2: From Dudek RW. *HY Cell and Molecular Biology*, 2nd ed. Baltimore: Lippincott Williams & Wilkins, 2007:104, Figure 12-3A–C.

Figure 1-3: From Dudek RW. *HY Cell and Molecular Biology*, 2nd ed. Baltimore: Lippincott Williams & Wilkins, 2007:91, Figure 10-2.

Figure 2-1: From Dudek RW. *HY Cell and Molecular Biology*, 2nd ed. Baltimore: Lippincott Williams & Wilkins, 2007:49–50, Figure 5-1. Original source: Reproduced with permission from Marks D. *BRS Biochemistry*, 3rd ed. Baltimore: Lippincott, Williams & Wilkins, 1999:46–47, Figures 3-1, 3-2, 3-3, 3-4.

Figure 2-2: **A.** From Dudek RW. *HY Cell and Molecular Biology*, 2nd ed. Baltimore: Lippincott Williams & Wilkins, 2007:51, Figure 5-2A. **B.** From Dudek RW. *HY Cell and Molecular Biology*, 2nd ed. Baltimore: Lippincott Williams & Wilkins, 2007:51, Figure 5-2B. Original source: Reprinted with permission of McKnight S, Miller OL. *Cell* 1976;8:305. **C.** From Dudek RW. *HY Cell and Molecular Biology*, 2nd ed. Baltimore: Lippincott Williams & Wilkins, 2007:51, Figure 5-2C.

Figure 3-1: From Dudek RW. *HY Cell and Molecular Biology*, 2nd ed. Baltimore: Lippincott Williams & Wilkins, 2007:42, Figure 4-2.

Figure 3-2: From Dudek RW. *HY Cell and Molecular Biology*, 2nd ed. Baltimore: Lippincott Williams & Wilkins, 2007:43, Figure 4-3.

Figure 4-1: From Dudek RW. *HY Cell and Molecular Biology*, 2nd ed. Baltimore: Lippincott Williams & Wilkins, 2007:6, Figure 8-2.

Figure 5-1: From Dudek RW, Fix JD. *BRS Embryology*, 3rd ed. Baltimore: Lippincott Williams & Wilkins, 2005:231, Figure 25-1.

Figure 5-2: **A.** From Swischuk LE. *Imaging of the Newborn, Infant, and Young Child*, 5th ed. Baltimore: Lippincott Williams & Wilkins, 2004:1097, Figure 7.159C. **B.** From Dudek RW, Louis TM. *HY Gross Anatomy*, 3rd ed. Baltimore: Lippincott Williams & Wilkins, 2008:76,

Figure 6-6A. Original source: Freundlich IM, Bragg DG. *A Radiologic Approach to Diseases of the Chest*, 2nd ed. Baltimore: Lippincott Williams & Wilkins, 1997:309, Figure 18-16. **C.** Dudek RW. *HY Histology*, 3rd ed. Baltimore: Lippincott Williams & Wilkins, 2004:113, Figure 11-3C. Original source: Stiene-Martin EA, Lotspeich-Steininger CA, Koepke JA. *Clinical Hematology: Principles, Procedures, and Correlations*, 2nd ed. Philadelphia: Lippincott Williams & Wilkins, 1998:96. **D.** McMillan JA et al. *Oski's Pediatrics: Principles and Practice*, 3rd ed. Baltimore: Lippincott Williams & Wilkins, 1999:1828, Figure 385-3A. **E.** McMillan JA, DeAngelis CD, Feigin RD, et al. *Oski's Pediatrics: Principles and Practice*, 3rd ed. Baltimore: Lippincott Williams & Wilkins, 1999:2004, Figure 414-1. **F.** McMillan JA et al. *Oski's Pediatrics: Principles and Practice*, 3rd ed. Baltimore: Lippincott Williams & Wilkins, 1999:248, Figure 37-5.

Figure 7-1: **A.** From Rubin R, Strayer DS, et al. *Rubin's Pathology*, 5th ed. Baltimore: Lippincott Williams & Wilkins, 2008:1266, Figure 29-22A. **B.** Rubin R, Strayer DS, et al. *Rubin's Pathology*, 5th ed. Baltimore: Lippincott Williams & Wilkins, 2008:1266, Figure 29-22B. **C.** Spitz JL. *Genodermatoses: A Full Color Clinical Guide to Genetic Skin Disorders*. Baltimore: Lippincott Williams & Wilkins, 1996:76, Figure 2-26. Courtesy of Lawrence Gordon, M.D., New York, NY. **D.** Dudek RW, Louis TM. *HY Gross Anatomy*, 3rd ed. Baltimore: Lippincott Williams & Wilkins, 2008: 52, Figure 5-2D. Original source: Daffner RH. *Clinical Radiology: The Essentials*, 2nd ed. Baltimore: Lippincott Williams & Wilkins, 1999:245, Figure 6-9. **E.** Dudek RW. *HY Histopathology*. Baltimore: Lippincott Williams & Wilkins, 2008:179, Figure 17-2B. Courtesy of R. W. Dudek, Ph.D. **F.** Rubin R, Strayer DS, et al. *Rubin's Pathology*, 5th ed. Baltimore: Lippincott Williams & Wilkins, 2008:607, Figure 13-58.

Figure 8-1: Dudek RW. *HY Embryology*, 3rd ed. Baltimore: Lippincott Williams & Wilkins, 2007:168, Figure 23-1F.

Figure 9-1: Dudek RW. *HY Cell and Molecular Biology*, 2nd ed. Baltimore: Lippincott Williams & Wilkins, 2007:127, Figure 15-2. Original source: Redrawn and modified with permission from Alberts et al. *Molecular Biology of the Cell*, 3rd ed. New York City: Garland Press, 1994.

Figure 9-2: Dudek RW. *HY Cell and Molecular Biology*, 2nd ed. Baltimore: Lippincott Williams & Wilkins, 2007:80–81, Figure 9-1A. Original sources: **A.** Dudek RW. *BRS Embryology*, 3rd ed. Baltimore: Lippincott Williams & Wilkins, 2005:2, Figure 1-1. **B.** Dudek RW.

BRS Embryology, 3rd ed. Baltimore: Lippincott Williams & Wilkins, 2005:3, Figure 1-2.

Figure 10-1: A. Courtesy of John E. Wiley, Ph.D. **B.** Dudek RW. *HY Cell and Molecular Biology*, 2nd ed. Baltimore: Lippincott Williams & Wilkins, 2007:52, Figure 5-3C. **C.** Courtesy of John E. Wiley, Ph.D. **D.** Modified from Westman JA. *Medical Genetics for the Modern Clinician*. Baltimore: Lippincott Williams & Wilkins, 2006:20, Figure 3-5. Courtesy of Dr. G. Wenger, Children's Hospital, Columbus, OH. **E.** Modified from Westman JA. *Medical Genetics for the Modern Clinician*. Baltimore: Lippincott Williams & Wilkins, 2006:20, Figure 3-5. Courtesy of Dr. Krzysztof Mrozek, The Ohio State University at Columbus, OH.

Figure 11-1: Dudek RW. *HY Embryology*, 3rd ed. Baltimore: Lippincott Williams & Wilkins, 2007:149, Figure 21-1.

Figure 11-2: Dudek RW. *HY Embryology*, 3rd ed. Baltimore: Lippincott Williams & Wilkins, 2007:161, Figure 22-3A.

Figure 11-3: A. Sadler TW. *Langman's Embryology*, 9th ed. Baltimore: Lippincott Williams & Wilkins, 2004:12, Figure 1-8B. **B.** Sadler TW. *Langman's Embryology*, 9th ed. Baltimore: Lippincott Williams & Wilkins, 2004:14, Figure 1-11. Original source: McKusick VA. Klinefelter and Turner's syndromes. *Journal of Chronic Disease* 1960;12:50. **C.** Nettina SM. *The Lippincott Manual of Nursing Practice*, 7th ed. Philadelphia: Lippincott Williams & Wilkins, 2001, Figure 56-2. **D.** McMillan JA et al. *Oski's Pediatrics: Principles and Practice*, 4th ed. Baltimore: Lippincott Williams & Wilkins, 2006:2638. **E.** Sadler TW. *Langman's Embryology*, 9th ed. Baltimore: Lippincott Williams & Wilkins, 2004:17, Figure 1-14. Courtesy of Dr. R. J. Gorlin, Department of Oral Pathology and Genetics, University of Minnesota. **F.** Sadler TW. *Langman's Embryology*, 9th ed. Baltimore: Lippincott Williams & Wilkins, 2004:16, Figure 1-13. Courtesy of Dr. R. J. Gorlin, Department of Oral Pathology and Genetics, University of Minnesota. **G.** Dudek RW. *HY Embryology*, 3rd ed. Baltimore: Lippincott Williams & Wilkins, 2007: 161, Figure 22-3C. Original source: Mufti GJ, Flandrin G. *An Atlas of Malignant Haematology*. Baltimore: Lippincott Williams & Wilkins, 1996:73,179. **H.** Dudek RW. *HY Embryology*, 3rd ed. Baltimore: Lippincott Williams & Wilkins, 2007:161, Figure 22-3D. Original source: Mufti GJ, Flandrin G. *An Atlas of Malignant Haematology*. Baltimore: Lippincott Williams & Wilkins, 1996:73,179. **I.** Spitz JL. *Genodermatoses*. Baltimore: Lippincott Williams & Wilkins, 1996:154, Figure 5-5. Courtesy of Gilles G. Lestringant, M.D., Abu Dhabi, United Arab Emirates. **J.** McMillan JA et al. *Oski's Pediatrics: Principles and Practice*, 3rd ed. Baltimore: Lippincott Williams & Wilkins, 1999: 2097, Figure 431-2.

Figure 13-1: Dudek RW. *HY Cell and Molecular Biology*, 2nd ed. Baltimore: Lippincott Williams & Wilkins, 2007:134, Figure 17-1.

Figure 13-3: A. Henrikson RC, Kaye GI, Mazurkiewicz JE. *NMS Histology*. Baltimore: Williams & Wilkins, 1999:104, Figure 8-4.

Figure 13-4: A. Dudek RW. *HY Heart*. Baltimore: Lippincott Williams & Wilkins, 2006:25, Figure 1-15A. Original source: Swischuk LE. *Imaging of the Newborn, Infant, and Young Child*, 5th ed. Baltimore: Lippincott Williams & Wilkins, 2004:298, Figure 3.108A. **B.** Stevens A, Lowe J. *Human Histology*, 2nd ed. London: Mosby, 1997:42, Figure 3-18. **C.** McMillan JA et al. *Oski's Pediatrics: Principles and Practice*, 4th ed. Baltimore: Lippincott Williams & Wilkins, 2006:2533, Figure 433-14A. **D.** Dudek RW, Fix J. *BRS Embryology*, 3rd ed. Baltimore: Lippincott Williams & Wilkins, 2005:178, Figure 17-1H. Original source: McMillan JA et al. *Oski's Pediatrics: Principles and Practice*, 3rd ed. Philadelphia: Lippincott Williams & Wilkins, 1999:396, Figure 66-9. Courtesy of M. M. Cohen Jr, Halifax, Nova Scotia, Canada. **E.** Spitz JL. *Genodermatoses: A Full Color Clinical Guide to Genetic Skin Disorders*. Baltimore: Lippincott Williams & Wilkins, 1996:151, Figure 5.1. Courtesy of Department of Dermatology, Columbia University, New York, NY. **F.** Dudek RW, Fix J. *BRS Embryology*, 3rd ed. Baltimore: Lippincott Williams & Wilkins, 2005:183, Figure 17-3G. Original source: McMillan JA et al. *Oski's Pediatrics: Principles and Practice*, 3rd ed. Philadelphia: Lippincott Williams & Wilkins, 1999:2149, Figure 433-8B. **G.** McMillan JA et al. *Oski's Pediatrics: Principles and Practice*, 4th ed. Baltimore: Lippincott Williams & Wilkins, 2006:2645. **H.** Dudek RW, Fix J. *BRS Embryology*, 3rd ed. Baltimore: Lippincott Williams & Wilkins, 2005:183, Figure 17-3E. Original source: McKusick VA. *Heritable Disorders of Connective Tissue*, 4th ed. St. Louis: CV Mosby, 1972:67. **I.** McMillan JA et al. *Oski's Pediatrics: Principles and Practice*, 4th ed. Baltimore: Lippincott Williams & Wilkins, 2006:2659. **J.** Swischuk LE. *Imaging of the Newborn, Infant, and Young Child*, 5th ed. Baltimore: Lippincott Williams & Wilkins, 2004:448, Figure 4-149B. **K.** Sadler TW. *Langman's Medical Embryology*, 9th ed. Baltimore: Lippincott Williams & Wilkins, 2004:394, Figure 15-29C. Courtesy of Dr. M. Edgerton, University of Virginia. **L.** McMillan JA et al. *Oski's Pediatrics: Principles and Practice*, 4th ed. Baltimore: Lippincott Williams & Wilkins, 2006:472, Figure 69-5.

Figure 14-1: A1. McMillan JA et al. *Oski's Pediatrics: Principles and Practice*, 4th ed. Baltimore: Lippincott Williams & Wilkins, 2006:2185, Figure 387-2. **A2.** Damjanov I. *Histopathology: A Color Atlas and Textbook*. Baltimore: Lippincott Williams & Wilkins, 1996:9, Figure 1-7A. **A3.** Damjanov I. *Histopathology: A Color Atlas and Textbook*. Baltimore: Lippincott Williams & Wilkins, 1996:9, Figure 1-7B. **B.** Damjanov I. *Histopathology: A Color Atlas and Textbook*. Baltimore: Lippincott Williams & Wilkins, 1996:454, Figure 18-4. **C.** Swischuk LE. *Imaging of the Newborn, Infant, and Young Child*, 5th ed. Baltimore: Lippincott Williams & Wilkins, 2004:1097, Figure 7-158B. **D.** Rubin R, Strayer DS, et al. *Rubin's Pathology*, 5th ed. Baltimore: Lippincott Williams & Wilkins, 2008:654, Figure 14-41. **E.** Damjanov I. *Histopathology: A Color Atlas and Textbook*. Baltimore: Lippincott Williams & Wilkins, 1996:10, Figure 1-9B. **F.** McMillan JA et al. *Oski's Pediatrics: Principles and Practice*, 4th ed. Baltimore: Lippincott Williams & Wilkins, 2006:2647. **G.** Sternberg SS et al. *Diagnostic Surgical Pathology*, Vol. 1, 4th ed. Baltimore:

Index

Note: Page numbers followed by f and t indicate figures and tables, respectively.